beauty fixes

beauty fixes

Everything you need to know about
'lunchtime' cosmetic treatments

JOSEPHINE FAIRLEY

Vermilion
LONDON

1 3 5 7 9 10 8 6 4 2

First published 2002 by Vermilion, an imprint of
Ebury Press · Random House
20 Vauxhall Bridge Road · London SW1V 2SA
www.randomhouse.co.uk

Random House Australia (Pty) Limited
20 Alfred Street · Milsons Point · Sydney
New South Wales 2061 · Australia

Random House New Zealand Limited
18 Poland Road · Glenfield · Auckland 10 · New Zealand

Random House South Africa (Pty) Limited
Endulini · 5a Jubilee Road · Parktown 2193 · South Africa

The Random House Group Limited Reg. No. 954009

A CIP catalogue record for this book is available from
the British Library.

ISBN 0 09 188223 0

Designed by Lovelock & Co.

Printed and bound in Great Britain by Bookmarque, Croydon, Surrey

Papers used by Vermilion are natural, recyclable products made
from wood grown in sustainable forests.

Contents

Introduction

We live in a time of fast food, speedy deliveries and blink-of-an-eye technology. An 'I-want-it-now' world. And where once the only option for someone wanting to turn back the clock was surgery, now there's a boom in cosmetic 'quick fixes': techniques which require less 'downtime' than cosmetic surgery but achieve more than creams, lotions and potions ever can. (Or are ever likely to: because cosmetic companies are now unable to do animal testing the way they used to, the beauty world won't be seeing as many revolutionary new ingredients in future, and must simply content itself with reformulating plant-and-science-based elements already in use.)

Certainly, in a world where appearances matter more than ever, women – and men – are refusing to age any faster than we have to. Where our mothers often embraced perms and cardigans at forty and gave up on feeling or looking like anything but dowdy mums (or grandmas), now we expect to look, and be, fabulous at forty/fifty/eighty, come to that. Hence the boom in BOTOX®, the craze for cosmetic peels – and the frenzy for 'filler' injections which make history of lines simply by, yes, filling them in.

They're often called 'lunchtime' procedures. But are they really? That's what you'll find out, from this book, which I wrote to help *you* work out the right procedure – if any – for you and your lifestyle. Ask a doctor, a clinic, a beauty therapist, and what you'll be told is inevitably a 'best-case scenario'. Your own recovery may be quite different – and it's important to be aware that some of these fixes aren't quite so quick in real life as they sound, requiring much more 'downtime' than simply taking an afternoon off while a touch of redness goes away. I've known women whose doctors have assured them they'll be back at their desks that same day – and who've ended up having to call in sick from work for a week while their bruises subside.

Of course it's up to you – not your sister, your husband or your best friend – to decide whether to have any of these procedures done. And I still believe it's worth trying everything else, first. So alongside information gathered from leading doctors, dermatologists and cosmetic surgeons in their fields, I've included tips in every chapter from top make-up artists and skin pros – as well as tricks I've learned in ten years as a beauty editor – for achieving many of the benefits of these cosmeto-dermatological methods in an entirely risk-free way. (Together with some ways of perhaps coming to terms with the 'you' that you see in the mirror.) I say: what have you got to lose by trying them? You may wind up saving yourself a small fortune in the process.

I felt that first-person case histories – from real people, who've raided their bank accounts to have these procedures done – were vital, too, to give the kind of this-is-how-it-is insight into BOTOX®/lasers/non-surgical facelifts that your best friend would share with you if *she'd* had it done. Because what's crucial, I believe, is to be armed with all the information you need to choose the right person, and the right procedure. Billions are being made by clinics, cosmeto-dermatologists (and even dentists, who carry out some of these rejuvenating techniques as a money-spinning sideline) out of this quest for enduring youth. None of these techniques is cheap; many of them require ongoing maintenance in order to keep up any benefits – for instance because the 'injectables' used are metabolised by the body over a period of months – and so represent a substantial investment.

And there can be a downside, as well as an upside. The pain factor. The cost factor. The 'botch' factor – because mistakes happen, particularly in the hands of inexperienced practitioners. The law of statistics says it's going to go wrong for *someone*. Murphy's Law says that could be *you*, if you don't take the savviest of approaches. As Dr Laurie Polis, one of Manhattan's leading cosmeto-dermatologists, told me when I interviewed her for this book, 'The risk may be a tiny, tiny percentage – but if it happens to you, it's a hundred per cent.'

The simple fact, meanwhile, is that there's no one-size-fits-all solution to the problems of ageing. Each of us is different – and successful treatment requires a tailor-made approach. As San Francisco dermatologist Dr Seth Matarasso explains: 'There is no one product for all seasons, for all patients or all doctors. Today, patients have many different options in the form of injectables, resurfacing and implant materials. You may find the best procedure to correct your facial lines and wrinkles is a combination of two or more of these – or that you really need laser or a facelift, instead.' However, that's a scenario that I truly hope this book will help you avoid.

What's legal also varies from country to country. But just because a product isn't approved for use in one particular country, that doesn't mean you can't find a doctor who'll do it for you. In the case of injectables, in particular, doctors go abroad and buy injectables that aren't available in their own country, and carry out the treatments with it back home.

I'm often asked: would I go in for this kind of cosmeto-dermatology, as it's called? I sometimes look in the mirror and dream of having my thread veins zapped – but I'm still at the stage of considering it, rather than booking my first appointment. Basically, I'm at ease in my (forty-five-year-old) skin. I like my laugh lines. I've been sensible enough to stay out of the sun most of my adult life, and am blessed with good genes – and yes, I do worry, long-term, about the potential side effects of some of these treatments. Is it *just* conceivable that BOTOX® – the toxin used to 'freeze' lines – might build up in the liver, if injected thrice-yearly, causing problems later? (Doctors assure me 'No, no, no', but that doesn't stop it niggling.

Because I'm sorry: it was the medical profession, after all, that reassured the British public there was no risk of the degenerative brain condition Creutzfeld-Jacob Disease from eating infected beef.) Could laser treatments one day turn out to trigger damage, deep in the skin? (Remember: once upon a time, we were told that sunbeds were perfectly safe...) Or could alpha-hydroxy acid peels – blitzing surface skin to reveal fresher, brighter layers underneath – leave the skin ultra-vulnerable to future damage, and so one day leave you looking older than if you'd left well alone? I wish I could tell you. But the bottom line is: nobody has those answers yet – because most of these procedures, in the grand scheme of things, are in their infancy. But they should all be on your list of questions to ask *yourself* if you're contemplating going under the laser/needle/layer of acid. Because then you'll be going into this with your eyes – as well as your chequebook – open.

One thing's for sure: quick fixes are here to stay. And whichever path you take – space-age or low-tech – I hope that this book helps you take the look-better decisions that will ensure you grow older gorgeously...

CHAPTER 1

Before you do a thing... how to find the best person for you

As with everything in life, some people are better at these techniques than others. In the case of a non-surgical facelift – in which the face is 'firmed' by stimulating the muscles with electrical currents – or a 'mega-facial', which I explore in the second half of this book, a trained beauty therapist will almost certainly be good enough for you to experience the best possible results. Many of the techniques in the first half of this book, though, require the expertise of a medical practitioner (and indeed, they may be the only people licensed to carry out this work).

My advice is: the more invasive and potentially risky the treatment, the more you want the reassurance that there's a doctor involved – if he's not giving you the treatment himself, then at least he's overseeing it, in case something goes wrong and you have a reaction or side effect that requires medical attention or advice. But interviewing the dozens of patients/clients for this book, I came across some who'd had nightmare results from a doctor – and some, by contrast, who raved about the skills of a beauty therapist who used BOTOX® or filler injections. The bottom line is: it's still a lottery, which is why you want to do as much homework as possible before you decide to place your face in anyone's hands.

Certainly, when these machines/procedures/fillers are initially launched, you tend only to find them carried out in a cosmetic surgeon's or a dermatologist's surgery. But as time goes by, beauty salons may see their business disappearing – which happened, in particular, in the case of laser hair removal; suddenly, people didn't want electrolysis any more. So the salon industry pushed to be allowed to be trained in the laser hair removal technology. (And does so, in most cases, very well.) Likewise filler injections, which I've heard of being administered by aestheticians who are definitely not trained nurses. At the moment, in the UK at least, the industry is awaiting greater regulation, which should come into force in around 2003 when the Standards of Care Bill becomes law, governing who can and cannot offer specific procedures and so safeguarding patient health.

Meanwhile: how do you find the right doctor/clinic/salon?

■ One of the very best recommendations is word of mouth.
  Perhaps the good news, then, is that having BOTOX® (or any of
  the other procedures in this book) has become so acceptable that
  the name of a good person is now used almost as social currency
  – I've overheard doctors' names being volunteered without
  anyone even asking for them! Don't be shy to ask around. The
  chances are, in this day and age, that a friend-of-a-friend knows
  someone who's had (whatever) done – and if they're pleased
  with the results, that's a good starting point. (By speaking to that
  person, you also gain inside information into how much it costs,
  how much it hurt and whether they were pleased with the
  results.) However, be aware that the procedure that worked for
  your friend may not be right for your face.

■ Consult the website of the association of plastic or cosmetic surgeons in your country (see RESOURCES) for a list of experts.

■ Consult an independent advisor. In an era when more and more people are opting for these techniques, independent consultants who can point you in the direction of the best possible person for you are going to become very busy indeed. It may be an extra layer of expense – you'll naturally have to pay for the consultation – but compared with the cost of most of these procedures, it's peanuts. It is also worth every penny if it saves you from a procedure that isn't right for you, or is badly performed. The woman who pioneered this is Wendy Lewis (see RESOURCES), who shuttles between New York and London, where she has practices, acting as an entirely independent consultant with no financial or professional ties to any doctors and clinics, and is therefore able to hand out entirely unbiased advice. (If ever there was a case for cloning, it's Wendy. There ought to be twenty of her.) She also has a great website packed with up-to-date information – and I consider her the 'fount of all wisdom' available on a one-to-one, specific-to-you basis. (I am also indebted to her for her extremely generous help with this book.)

Be aware, though, that some clinics set themselves up to sound like an independent advisor – calling themselves 'Advisory Services' or 'So-And-So Clinic' – but are actually a front for just one surgeon, not independent at all. You meet with a so-called 'advisor', believing they're going to help you pinpoint the right procedure and doctor for you within the clinic's portfolio of professionals – whereas in fact, there's only one doctor there. If you do go to a 'medical centre' or 'advisory centre', be sure there's more than one person administering treatments or doing surgery.

■ You could try asking your general practitioner to refer you to a cosmeto-dermatologist – but you'll probably get short shrift as most of these are filed under 'vanity' in an NHS doctor's mind. And be aware that your family doctor probably won't know either the best person for you to go to, or the most appropriate techniques.

■ My advice is: don't just blindly follow up an advertisement in a glossy magazine or newspaper and don't imagine that whoever is advertising is the best person or clinic around. In my experience, the very best people don't advertise – because word of mouth brings them more work than they can reasonably handle; most have waiting lists and you should consider this a good sign. While some of the clinics and doctors that advertise may well be perfectly competent, this can also be where problems occur – with unqualified staff actually carrying out procedures, and/or poor facilities. However, if there is absolutely no way for you to access this kind of technique other than by following up an advertisement, and you are convinced that a 'quick fix' is for you (having weighed up all the advice in this book), then approach several clinics and/or doctors who advertise, not just one, so that you have a point of comparison. Be thorough in your questioning. (See VITAL QUESTIONS TO ASK opposite.) Compare what they tell you and choose a surgeon or practitioner with whom you feel you have a rapport and can trust.

■ Above all, be extremely wary of 'visiting' practitioners who travel around the country carrying out procedures in places like hotels and beauty salons. As Vancouver-based Dr Alastair Carruthers observes, 'I am staggered at the way some people allow themselves to be injected by strangers who travel from place to place, setting up temporary shop. Some of the worst catastrophes I've seen resulted from treatments carried out in these circumstances. The more you can do in the way of background checks, the better.' Advises Wendy Lewis: 'These "Have BOTOX®, will travel" doctors are often GPs trying to get around stringent

NHS regulations that do not allow them to treat their own patients privately.'

■ Some beauty clinics or cosmetic surgeons arrange demonstrations to promote their techniques to groups of women or members of ladies' clubs. This is fraught with pitfalls. If the person who'll be giving the treatment is just passing through town (see above), they may do a disappearing act on you – leaving you with no redress if the treatment goes wrong. And the demonstrations themselves can be something of a con. As one representative for a manufacturer of filler injections – who for obvious reasons wished to remain nameless – told me, 'You may see fabulous results on a patient before your very eyes. But ask questions about the quantity of filler used, and ask how that compares to what you'd have injected in a typical treatment. I've seen demos where the amount of filler used was four or five times what the average patient would receive per injection – so the real cost would be much, much more expensive than you've been quoted.'

Vital questions to ask

Amazingly, there are people who sign up for some of the medical procedures featured in this book without giving them much more thought than if they were out shopping for a new face cream. If we buy a 'miracle cream' that doesn't suit us, though, we just throw it away and start slapping on something else instead. When you've had a 'filler' injection, or your complexion's been virtually sandblasted, you have to live with the results for months. Or longer. (Some of the 'fillers' – for instance SoftForm™, Artecoll® and Evolution – are permanent. And I've certainly known of one case where a 'filler' was used on a young-ish, plump-ish face – with perfect results – but those lines actually turned into obvious ridges as that face aged and slimmed down and the filler became visible on the thinner surface.)

For all of the procedures in Chapters 3–8, you want to ask some serious questions before you hand over a penny. In every instance, you should insist on a preliminary consultation in which to discuss whether the technique is right for you – allowing yourself enough time to go away and mull it over before committing. (Otherwise you wouldn't be the first person who's been cowed into having something done that they've actually had second thoughts about – but were too shy to walk out.) So...

1   Make an appointment with one or two doctors/clinics (or, where appropriate, salons) for an initial consultation. You may well find there's a fee for this, which is sometimes deducted from the fee for the procedure if you decide to go ahead. (If you don't decide to go ahead, you should still consider the money well spent, invested in ensuring that you don't make a mistake.) Try to insist on meeting the person who'll actually be carrying out the procedure – not his right-hand woman/man, because that's the important relationship here.

2   Tap into your intuition: how do you get along with the person who's going to be wielding the needle/laser/whatever? This is someone you should feel you can trust. Discuss the different options with them – and listen to your heart and instincts. If you feel at any stage that you're the object of a marketing/sales operation, that person is probably more interested in his fee than in you, the would-be patient.

3   Ask for detailed information on the procedures you're thinking about. Many surgeons provide their own fact sheets, and may carry a wealth of literature from the suppliers of the fillers/equipment they use. Ask about any possible complications, the pain factor – and what relief will be available to you – as well as recovery times. Be aware that no honest

surgeon can guarantee a specific result – we are all individuals.
(So be wary of anyone who does…) Questions to ask are:

- In the case of filler injections, 'What is the source of the material?' (Animal/synthetic etc. – some fillers actually come from human foreskins, or are donated tissue from dead bodies.) 'Then you can make up your mind whether you want it inside your body,' advises Wendy Lewis.
- 'How long will the implant/procedure last?' (This helps you decide whether you can afford the maintenance.)
- 'How many treatments will I need for full correction?'
- 'How much will each treatment cost? Does that include follow-up visits?'
- 'What are the risks and possible side effects? How common are they?'
- 'Given my skin type, what results can I expect?'
- 'Can I have an allergic reaction? Is a skin test required before treatment?'
- 'What if I don't like it? (i.e. 'Is the procedure reversible, will it fade in time – and will it be repeated at no charge to me?')
- 'What is the maintenance if I want to keep the effects up, and what will the cost of those be?'
- 'How will I look immediately after the treatment? Is it realistic that I will be able to go back to work or out to dinner immediately afterwards?'

4 Most importantly, ask to see photographs of patients who've had this procedure/technique carried out by this specific doctor/aesthetician. (I have heard of instances where some unscrupulous doctors have shown the handiwork of colleagues, or from the laser manufacturer's own literature, rather than their own.) Do remember that you'll never be shown the worst results – only the best. Try to see a patient in person who's successfully

had the treatment you're interested in. (Although be aware that usually these will be the clinic staff, who tend to act as resident 'guinea pigs' for the procedures the doctor carries out.)

5   In the same way, it's perfectly legitimate to ask to speak to someone who's had the procedure carried out at this location, by this person. (Many people find this very reassuring.)

6   Check out the doctor's/nurse's/aesthetician's qualifications and training. Ask him/her which professional bodies he/she is a member of, and for the phone number of those bodies. If you have the slightest niggle, you can ring them to confirm. (As one doctor told me, 'Believe it or not, some unscrupulous doctors do lie about their qualifications.')

7   Ask if the surgeon/clinic is comprehensively insured.

8   Have a good look around before you leave. Is the place clean? Does he/she employ professional-seeming assistants and nurses? It's a fact that good doctors tend to attract good staff. Don't be taken in by plush carpets and flashy portraits on the wall; ask to see inside the room where the rejuvenating technique will take place, and satisfy yourself that it is all that you would hope a clinical environment to be. (I've seen some surprisingly grubby and shabby places.) You may also want to satisfy yourself that there's somewhere private for you to sit and recover emotionally, if you need to – rather than returning to the waiting room alongside other patients.

9   Beware of a surgeon who seems over-eager to treat you, or offers to do it the next day, who claims to be the only doctor qualified to do the procedure, doesn't mention risks or offers cut-price procedures. (However tempting that may seem.)

10 Before you leave the consultation, feel comfortable that you have a clear understanding of the possible procedures, the risk and recovery times. Ask for those details in writing – plus a written quotation for the precise costs and number of follow-up visits. Be sure you are aware what the 'maintenance' is on each procedure, so that you can be sure you can afford any upkeep. Do listen carefully to what the doctor or aesthetician is saying. A patient/client with unrealistic expectations may end up going back for procedure after procedure, perhaps making a problem worse instead of better.

What your doctor/salon needs to know about you

Asking is only half the story. Sharing your own details – about lifestyle, medical records, skincare regime and more – is also vital to ensure the best possible chance of a successful treatment. When things do go wrong, it's sometimes because of non-disclosure on the part of the patient/client, resulting in an adverse reaction that could have been avoided if you were cross-your-heart-and-hope-to-die 100 per cent truthful.

Wherever there's an 'action', there's always a possibility – however slight – of a 'reaction'. You can play a really crucial role in reducing your risk by providing a full and complete health history. This includes:

- Any medications you may be taking of any kind – even over-the-counter medicines.
- Any vitamin supplements that you are taking.
- Any history of blood pressure or heart problems, lung problems or diseases of the central nervous system, as well as cancer, diabetes and any auto-immune diseases. (If you know you are HIV-positive or have/carry hepatitis A, B or C, you must of course communicate this, too.)

- Vulnerability to heat and sunburn, or light-sensitive conditions (such as porphyria or Polymorphic Light Eruption).
- Allergies – however irrelevant they may seem, including hay fever and food intolerances. (Some fillers, for instance, are unsuitable for patients with an allergy to eggs.)
- Sensitivity to cosmetics and skin creams.
- How badly you bruise. If you know you go black and blue easily, tell your doctor/nurse. As one distributor of filler injections told me, 'Some doctors will whack the stuff in. If you tell them that you bruise easily, they can go more gently.'

This may, to you, be the boring part of the consultation. But it might make the difference between walking out of there smiling. Or (for whatever reason) sobbing.

Now think about it...

Only fools rush in – and you should avoid any clinic that pressurises you to make a decision immediately. So sleep on it. Talk to your friends/partner about it. (You may find that the person you live with, or your children, are vehemently opposed to the idea because they love you just the way you are. And while you may think you'll be able to have it done and nobody will notice, as I've already explained, some of the procedures don't turn out to be 'lunchtime fixes' at all.)

If you do opt to have the treatment, you'll be asked to sign a consent form. Read every word before flourishing your signature on the dotted line – and be aware that the consent form is actually designed to protect the surgeon, the medical system and the manufacturers, rather than you. If you sign the consent form, that implies that all the risk and possible complications have been spelled out to you – and that you understand them. So if you're unsure about something, ask for clarification before you sign.

CHAPTER 2

Acceptance...

When I started this book, I hadn't a clue what the motivations of the women I'd find for my case histories might turn out to be. A desperate quest for lost youth? An attempt to regain the attention of a husband whose eyes (or hands) were straying? Or simply an attempt to keep up, in an increasingly lookist world?

Boy, was I about to be surprised. Almost without exception, the dozens of women I met and spoke to were doing this for themselves – the same way they'd invest in a good suit, a great haircut, or colour their hair to cover the grey. It was a matter of self-respect – not clutching at straws, in any way. In just a couple of years, these 'cosmetic tweaks', these 'quick fixes', the 'lunchtime procedures' – call them what you like, have gone from taboo to 100 per cent socially acceptable, in many circles.

Without exception, I promised my case histories anonymity, to encourage full disclosure of the upside *and* the downside of their experiences. But to my amazement, about half of them insisted that no, it was fine to print their full name; they didn't mind *who* found out they were having this stuff done. In the end, for the sake of consistency, I stuck to a first name and an age for everyone – just as I'd promised to the women who did want to keep their secret. (Who were, in case you're wondering, almost without exception the older interviewees.)

Nonetheless, as the quick fix becomes more acceptable – and infinitely more accessible – I still think it's important to ask yourself, before you go ahead with many of the procedures in the first half of this book, *why* you want to have it done. Is it simply to be the best that you can? A matter of self-esteem? Or, just possibly, because you hope that, somehow, the procedure will wave a magic wand – or a magic laser – over other problems in your life?

When I edited women's magazines, our postbag bulged with letters from readers who believed that getting their nose fixed or their boobs enhanced would land them the perfect job/man/flat. It won't, we assured them. Quite often, they'd ignore our 'agony aunt's' advice and go ahead and get their noses/chin/breasts fixed. Those same women would often be back in touch, six months later: 'I now think that maybe I should have liposuction, because I'm still not happy...' For those in constant quest of perfection, psychologists have even coined a name: 'excessorexics'. As Dr Derek Roger of York University (who's carried out research into the syndrome) observes: 'The world is changing, and people today feel under pressure to be successful and generally portray a perfect image to the rest of the world. There's an ethos that feeds this perfectionism because now we believe that nothing is ever good enough. What people don't realise is that much of the pressure comes from internal forces – it doesn't really exist at all.'

Certainly, it rapidly became clear to me while compiling the interviews that the first 'quick fix' is the hardest. Once you've had one procedure – well, why not another, and another? A shot of Botulinum Toxin in the forehead. A red vein or two zapped. And maybe a plumper lip... Many of the women I spoke to, once they'd broken through the mental barrier of having their first BOTOX® or collagen, readily admitted to being 'hooked' – with all the investment of time and money that entails.

So before you start on that path, I think it's worth trying the 'acceptance' route...

■ Look in the mirror and analyse the lines on your face in repose. Smile, and look again. Think of the positive emotions that put some of those lines there: happiness, joy, laughter. Do you really want to erase that from your appearance? Are there ways to put more joy in your life? (Fact: nobody who's smiling looks old…) What would you like to be doing more of in your life – gardening, travelling, spending time with friends? Maybe it's time to do more of that, and less of whatever it is that gives you the frown-lines.

■ And about those frown-lines: could getting your eyes tested – or buying a new pair of sunglasses – help that problem? Are there annoyances in your life that could be simply solved – or could finding a way of bringing down your overall stress level help?

■ How much time each day do you devote to worrying about your appearance – above and beyond maintenance, cleanliness and general good grooming? Are there other positive channels for that time and energy – doing something for your soul, like meditation or yoga, or going for a walk in nature? (Because you'll probably also find that has a knock-on benefit for your appearance, too.)

■ Do the people around you love and like you the way you are? Because if so, what are you worrying about? (And if they don't, should you be thinking of updating your address book – not your face?)

■ Are you considering this because everyone else you know is having something done, because it's 'the fashion' – and you're worried about being left out? If I may be so bold, that's a rubbish reason.

■ Dr Roger also suggests altering your mind-set before excessorexia sets in. 'Try to understand and accept the real you,' he advises. 'You aren't defined by your clothes, your body, your job or your possessions. Don't impose standards on your life that aren't real. If you do, you will lead a miserable life, because you will never be perfect enough.'

■ Meanwhile, have you tried all the insider tricks and techniques – and the products – that might be able to achieve some of the results of the procedures you're considering, so saving you time and money on doctor's appointments? (Find them in the CHEATS section at the end of each chapter, and try them before you dial that doc...)

Personally, I believe that the ageing process is called life. It's what happens. As we age, there are changes and to a certain extent we have to go with the flow, because the trade-off – of *who* we are inside – is worth a wrinkle or two. We'd all love to look the way we were and be the way we were – but that isn't realistic. So we have to come to terms with imperfection. The balance has to shift: instead of the emphasis being on the physical, we have to develop an inner life to draw on, shifting the focus to values and quality of life. (Because if we aren't careful, focussing on the physical can become an obsession.)

As Leslie Kenton, guru of the natural approach to beauty, observes, 'I'd say to anyone who was considering a procedure first to take up weight training, look at your insulin levels, lower the carbohydrate in your diet and eat lots of salad and green vegetables. Neurotransmitters, the hormones in our brain that control feelings, are derived from the food we eat, so our diet needs to be good if we want to be in excellent mental health – to feel good about ourselves.' She reckons that after six months of following her prescription for healthier living – which she's written down in book after readable, brilliant book – most women won't *want* to mess with their faces or bodies.

And if you try all that and still feel you need extra help to be the best that you can be? Then this book should arm you with everything you need to help ensure that your 'quick fix' is one of the successes – not one of the disasters...

CHAPTER 3

BOTOX® – the line tamer

BOTOX®. Or, to give it its full name, Botulinum Toxin. Get any group of women together and it probably won't be long before the conversation turns to BOTOX®: 'Have you had it?' 'Would you have it?' 'What's it like?' (Personally, scanning a room for foreheads that look like they've been ironed has become something of a sport for me.)

So I feel that BOTOX® deserves a chapter all of its own – because quite frankly, it's sweeping the world like a wanna-look-good pandemic. There are even women holding BOTOX® 'parties', where a rent-a-doc will come and inject a group of friends somewhere between the rocket salad, the sea bass and the Ben'n'Jerry's ice cream.

An injection – of a highly poisonous toxin (albeit in the teeniest of quantities) – BOTOX® has the effect of 'freezing' (for which read: paralysing) muscles, so that they can no longer make certain expressions, particularly frowning or squinting. 'If you look at elderly stroke victims with partial facial paralysis,' says Dr Patricia Wexler, leading New York dermatologist and one of BOTOX®'s foremost 'gurus', 'you'll notice that the paralysed side is completely wrinkle-free. It's the same principle at work with BOTOX®.' Originally used in medicine to treat conditions like muscle spasm and Bell's Palsy, its use as an anti-wrinkle treatment was stumbled upon by Dr Alastair Carruthers, a Vancouver-based skin doctor – or rather, his wife Jean.

An eye doctor who'd been using it to treat tics, her patients began telling her that their wrinkles were improved. Dr Carruthers experimented – and now, it's the hottest 'cosmetic tweak' on the menu.

Look out, too, for a new-generation BOTOX® coming down the (facial) line: Myobloc® (marketed as Neuroblock® in the UK). Until recently only used to stop spasms associated with neurological problems, it was only a matter of time before some savvy doctor started using it to treat wrinkles – and sure enough, it's happened. Myobloc® is available in a strong, ready-to-use solution – which means that (unlike with BOTOX® 'original') doctors who want to cut corners can't over-dilute it. But Myobloc® is not without problems, even at this stage: according to Dr Wexler, Myobloc® 'has been associated with dry mouth and difficulty swallowing'.

What worries women I've spoken to is the potential risk, years down the line, of BOTOX® being stored in the body – and ultimately, when you've had the shots three or four times a year for twenty-something age-defying years, of it causing serious health problems. They worry about cancer, in particular, or neurological diseases. Well, Dr Carruthers is quite reassuring on that front. 'We use absolutely tiny quantities, injected into the muscle – not the bloodstream,' he says. Because BOTOX® has been in medical use for twenty years, he says, they'd know by now if it caused longer-term problems. (And certainly, as independent cosmetic surgery consultant and self-confessed BOTOX® junkieWendy Lewis observes, 'BOTOX® is the single procedure most often carried out by cosmetic doctors on themselves, and their families.') The fact is that if you ask whether there are potentially any long-term health risks, doctors will invariably insist: 'No' – and the long-term studies simply don't exist. (But you should at least be asking yourself: what if...? before you make that appointment...)

Now, call me a worry-wort, but I still fret: the body's way of dealing with toxins is to store them in the liver: the body's giant filtration plant. As someone who eats (almost exclusively) organic food because I'm concerned not only about the planet but my own future health, I'm not about to have myself injected with this stuff. End of story. But you have to make up your own mind. There are millions of happy, smooth-browed BOTOX®-lovers – as well as, some people who have personal disaster stories to tell, having wound up with drooping eyebrows or an angry expression that took months to wear off. I've included several first-person case histories – male and female – so that you can gauge for yourself what the results may be.

If you decide you're interested, follow the guidelines in the beginning of this book to find your BOTOX® doctor, ask all the right questions and be sure you go into it with your eyes open. BOTOX® is meant to be carried out by trained medical practitioners – i.e. doctors and nurses. However, according to Dr Alastair Carruthers, this is so abused that he's even come across a patient who was injected by her doctor's wife: 'She couldn't open her eye afterwards, because the BOTOX® was injected in the wrong place.' Reassure yourself that the person who you choose for your BOTOX® treatment is adequately qualified – and insured. Preferably, find someone who's done this thousands and thousands of times – and be aware that even good doctors have bad days.

BOTOX®

The low-down A safe derivative of deadly botulism bacteria is injected into the expression lines, paralysing the muscle. The effect isn't immediate and 'kicks in' after somewhere between three to eight days as the treated muscles gradually weaken. (The timing varies from patient to patient.) When the muscle reflex is lost, the wrinkle or crease goes away. (Some doctors apply a numbing cream before BOTOX®, some don't. Find out, and if you want one, say so.) As with so many fillers, success rests on the skill of the dermatologist, who dilutes the BOTOX® to the concentration he or she believes is required, and then gauges the best dose: 100 per cent correction of crow's feet may leave a face mask-like.

Suitable for Men and women with frown and squint lines, like the folds between the eyebrows, vertical or horizontal folds on the forehead and crow's feet. (BOTOX® is also now being used as a treatment for excessive sweating, although I won't be covering that aspect in this book.) Some extremely experienced doctors – including Miami-based Dr Fredric Brandt, the 'king' of BOTOX® (who uses more of the stuff than any single other surgeon) – are now pioneering a BOTOX® 'neck-lift', injecting the substance into the 'cords' around the neck that can emerge as we age.

Not suitable for BOTOX® is never used around the mouth, where 'freezing' would be aesthetically unacceptable; drooling is one possible side effect. According to Professor Nicholas Lowe, Clinical Professor at UCLA School of Medicine, and Consultant Dermatologist at The Cranley Clinic, London and Santa Monica. 'It should not be used to treat the lower half of the face as it can cause muscle droop.' BOTOX® injections can't be used in pregnancy, or when breast-feeding.

Recovery time BOTOX® really is a 'lunchtime fix'; most people who are injected go straight back to work or to a social engagement. Some people have a slight headache after treatment; if so, it's safe to take paracetamol. A small bruise at the site of injection is also fairly common. It's important to remain upright for at least an hour after you have a BOTOX® shot, and although you can frown as often as you like, you should definitely avoid any kind of facial massage.

The risks There is a small risk of redness or swelling at the site of injection. Although allergy to BOTOX® is said to be impossible, Dr Alastair Carruthers observes: 'The BOTOX® injection contains human serum albumen and in a tiny, tiny percentage of cases – perhaps 1 per cent – there may be a mild, hive-like reaction or flu-like symptoms, which are a reaction to the albumen, not the toxin itself.' According to Vincent Longo, a make-up artist who's seen many recently injected BOTOX® patients up-close-and-personal, 'The worst reaction I saw was a serious case of redness, almost blistering – although this went away in a couple of days.' The most common significant complication, which is rare, is called 'ptosis'; this is a drooping of the eyelid caused by the botulinum toxin travelling into the eyelid muscle; it generally lasts just a few days, but a longer weakness is possible. (Your doctor can prescribe eye drops that will lessen this effect.) As you'll see from the case histories that follow, there's also a risk of the eyebrows drooping if the BOTOX® is wrongly injected. There is occasionally talk, too, of patients who are (or who become) 'immune' to BOTOX® – but Dr Carruthers believes this can very often be put down to 'operator error' – in other words, the doctor didn't administer the BOTOX® into the correct muscle, use enough of the toxin, or may have over-diluted it. 'I like to see patients two weeks after treatment, to check the results,' he says. (It's worth pressing for this with your own doctor.) I've heard cautionary tales of unnaturally frozen faces – but when I tried to find someone for this book who'd suffered this problem, they proved as elusive as, well, the Loch Ness monster or fairies at the bottom of the garden. (Feel free to e-mail me, however, at quickfixes@josephinefairley.com, if it's happened to you or someone you know.) But not everyone's happy with the results – as you'll see from Penny's story on page 34.

Upkeep Results should last from three to six months. Some patients report that they become so unfamiliar with their paralysed muscles that they literally 'forget' how to flex them, even after the effect has worn off – rendering the effects of BOTOX® much more permanent.

How much it costs From approximately £200 per treated area.

'I had BOTOX® to combat ageing'

– JANICE, 56

'My first husband passed away seven years ago and a couple of years later, I hooked up with an old boyfriend who was working in my home town of Vancouver. We fell in love all over again and got engaged. I now often find myself in the role of playing hostess to his business colleagues. I don't want to look like a goddess, but I want to look the best I possibly can. It's about being your personal best. And besides, what bride doesn't want to look as good as possible?

'I do not have a "shopping-mall mentality" and tend to align myself with good physicians; I wouldn't do anything I hadn't read about and researched, or go to someone I heard about from a girlfriend at lunch. (In fact, I've never really had the time for lunches!) Whenever needles are involved, of course there are also fears about HIV transmission, so I needed to feel completely confident in the ability of my doctor. I've never had any kind of cosmetic dermatology before BOTOX®, although I do see a dermatologist for general skin health. (I am fair, and I have a time-share in Mexico, so I've had a fair bit of sun exposure over the years. It's only sensible to keep an eye open for any changes to moles.) I have seen friends have facelifts and been fairly horrified by what they cost; I also don't like what I see – in some, the jawline looks really unnatural afterwards. I believe that doctors have to have a good aesthetic sense; the way our faces move is integral to our personality, and so the physician has to have a sensitivity to the whole person as an individual. He can't be a mechanic. I would consider my doctor, Dr Carruthers, a true artist.

'I had my BOTOX® treatment sitting semi-reclined in the chair. Each injection – there are several – was like a short, biting jab; I could barely feel anything. Initially, there's no sign of any change – not even a needle-mark, in my case. But over eight or ten days, the BOTOX® took hold and it was as if my face was being gradually ironed out. I didn't have very obvious frown-lines or horizontal lines on my forehead, but afterwards, the area just looked super-smooth – and so, as a result, much more youthful. It doesn't feel in any way strange; you're not conscious of not being able to move those muscles. The effect lasts for around three months before gradually, almost imperceptibly, the lines start to re-emerge and it's time for a top-up. I feel this is one of the best-researched treatments around, with a huge amount of research into the effects. For me, a quick trip to the dermatologist's office every three months or so is the perfect low-maintenance, high-return, anti-ageing tactic.'

CASE STUDY

'I had BOTOX® to prevent wrinkles'

– MICHAEL, 37

'Lots of men I know are going for BOTOX® now – it's the natural extension of becoming more interested in fitness and grooming; in fact, 30 per cent of the patients the doctor from whom I had my treatment sees are now male. In reality, I don't have that many wrinkles but I was told that BOTOX® could also work to prevent expression lines from forming – and that appealed to me. I liked the fact that it wasn't permanent, so I didn't feel threatened; if I didn't like how it looked or felt, then in four or five months it would have gone and I'd be back to "me". First of all, the doctor asked me to contort my face so he could see my where lines were likely to form, and then he made little dots along them with a marker; that's where the injections were to go.

'The BOTOX® paste was mixed with water and then injected, which stung slightly. It was a little uncomfortable but not screamingly painful on the forehead, yet it didn't hurt at all around the eyes. (Apparently women have a much higher pain threshold than men and so find it more bearable.) He injected using several small injections in a "V" shape on my forehead, and then used another three small injections on either eye; at the end, there was still plenty of BOTOX® left in the syringe. There was a small red mark where the needle had gone in but this was gone by morning. A girlfriend who came with me for a BOTOX®

treatment at the same time simply covered hers up with powder. Certainly, there was no bruising – and I bruise terribly easily; if I bang into a chair I go as black and blue as if I've been beaten up. The whole process took twelve minutes – I timed it.

'I spent the next few days excitedly dashing to the mirror to see if I could make out any change but it creeps up on you very slowly, between the fourth and sixth day. I felt like it had really smoothed out my skin – almost as if it had been "ironed". When it first starts to "kick in" you're incredibly conscious of it, and I spent quite a lot of time trying to make expressions – and being unable to. It feels like you're frowning or raising an eyebrow – not at all as if your face is immobile – but your reflection simply isn't making those faces. But if you touch your skin, it still has all sensation – not like a dental injection, when you can't feel anything. The lack of movement does feel a bit alien – but you adjust so rapidly to the sensation that after a few days, it's as if it's always been like that. The only problem is: I can't do irony any more! I think I'm raising my eyebrows at something a friend's said – and they're just getting a blank stare!'

CASE STUDY 'I had BOTOX® for my frown-lines'

– PAULETTE, 42

'I am a squinter. I'm always losing my glasses or peering at things – and as a result, at forty, I've developed two frown-lines running vertically between my brows. A friend suggested BOTOX® – and pointed me in the direction of a very experienced medical doctor who treats patients with it.

'An anaesthetic cream was applied to my forehead to numb it. And then he did two injections, one into each frown-line. I have a very low pain threshold, but there was absolutely no "ouch" factor. I thought that it would feel weird afterwards, and that my brow might be numb – rather like what happens to your lip when you go to the dentist. But I wasn't conscious at all of the fact that I couldn't now frown; it happened gradually over a week and I didn't feel paralysed. It just felt very natural.

'I was told that it would last around three months – and it did, almost. During that time, my forehead looked smoother and I suppose I looked a little younger – or maybe less cross! – but I can't say that it made a dramatic difference. Even my husband didn't notice. So to be honest, I'm not going to have it done again. The upkeep seems like a lot of bother. And I'd rather invest the money in a couple of spare pairs of spectacles.'

CASE STUDY 'I had NeuroBloc® – because BOTOX® failed'

– PAULA, 33

'I had BOTOX® a year ago – as a birthday present to myself – and for four months it was fantastic. I had it for fine lines and wrinkles on my forehead, between my brows and around my eyes. I'm around the age women start to develop these fine lines, and basically I didn't want them to get any worse. I work as a nurse and I'd read a lot about BOTOX®, and my overriding impression was that it was very safe, because it's been so widely used not only as an anti-ageing treatment but therapeutically in medicine.

'BOTOX® worked perfectly the first time, so when I went back for my top-up after four months I had high expectations. The first time it had kicked in after two days – but the second time, although it was quite effective on my frown-lines for about a month, the horizontal lines on my forehead and my laugh-lines didn't "freeze" at all – which was hugely disappointing. My doctor, Dr Patrick Bowler, explained that in a very few cases, patients are resistant to BOTOX® – and I was one of the unlucky few. He gave me another free top-up – and this time, it didn't work at all. But he did say that he'd recently been at a medical conference where Myobloc® – or Botulinum Toxin B – was discussed, and that he hoped to start using it before long.

'About six months later, he got back in touch and told me that he was now using Myobloc® – which is marketed as NeuroBloc® in the UK. I couldn't wait to see if it worked. I found that the injections stung a bit more than BOTOX® – and basically, you can't get around that by applying a local anaesthetic because the injection goes to a deeper level in the skin than would be numbed by a local. So I put up with the stinging, and quite a lot of pressure – nothing intolerable, just a bit uncomfortable. (It was worse between the eyebrows; not so bad around the eyes or the forehead.)

'Whereas the original BOTOX® "took" after about two days, it was six before NeuroBloc® took effect – which had me wondering whether I was resistant to this, too. Then my face started to look more relaxed – almost as if the lines had been "ironed" – and I realised, yes, it had worked. It doesn't stop me smiling with my eyes, but it does stop me frowning, which is a good thing. What I do believe, though, is that as with any cosmetic procedure, it's vital to find the right doctor. Working in medicine I know that there are cowboys out there, and I don't want just anyone messing with my face. That's the advice I'd give to my girlfriends – who are all keen to have BOTOX® sooner or later, but are mostly put off by the cost. As time goes on, though, and there's more competition, these procedures are becoming cheaper.

'NeuroBloc® seems to work for me where BOTOX® failed, and I'll continue to have my top-ups. Maybe nobody would notice my wrinkles – any more than they'd notice if I broke out in a spot – but I do. And ironing out my lines in this way just makes me feel better about myself.'

CASE STUDY   'My BOTOX® was a nightmare'

– PENNY, 53

'I have had a frown-mark since the age of ten. As a little girl, I was always told not to frown, but I did it automatically – and the mark's the result. I've tried sleeping with sticky tape on it and trying to be conscious of not frowning – but to no avail. I knew someone else who'd had BOTOX® and it looked terrific; she'd had such good results, I decided to give it a try. I did all the right things – called up the governing body of plastic surgeons – and found a proper doctor.

'I went along and was told it would be very easy to rectify the line. I signed all the appropriate consent forms, and then the treatment went ahead. The doctor told me, though, that he would only give me half the usual dose because it was my first time – and if I wanted more, after the results became clear in three days, then I could come back for a top-up. A numbing cream was rubbed in and I was injected just above the eyebrow, either side. It was a little swollen afterwards, but nothing significant. After three days, I felt the line was about 50 per cent gone – but for me, that wasn't enough; I expected to see a smooth forehead, so I made another appointment.

'What the doctor observed was that in fact, the BOTOX® had effectively removed the centre area of the horizontal lines across my forehead, rather than the vertical line that really bothers me. He said he didn't want to give me more BOTOX® in the line I disliked, but that he'd give me a bit more to make the other, horizontal lines disappear – even though those lines don't really trouble me. I went through the same procedure. Then three days later, when the BOTOX® kicked in, my eyebrows drooped. I had read that a small percentage of people have a bad result, but I somehow never expected it to be me. I felt it changed my face completely and for the three months that the BOTOX® lasted, I couldn't do anything about it. My eyebrow didn't have a natural arch – and I couldn't raise my brows even if I tried. My eyes were half-closed and I just looked a combination of half-asleep and thunderously cross, until it gradually wore off. All that time, people commented how tired I looked or said, "Cheer up!" I was really upset, even though it may not have looked as bad to other people as it did to me.

'I took it as a warning and decided that I would never, ever have anything done like that again. From now on, I will be growing old gracefully.'

BOTOX®: The cheats

■ According to leading international hairstylist John Frieda, 'If you have a furrowed or lined forehead, you should try a fringe before you try anything else. A fringe over the brow can be extremely de-ageing for older women, softening a face and even disguising lines. Steer clear of heavy fringes, though, as this look is too severe for women of practically any age. Go for something light and feathery.'

■ If you have a vertical line/lines between the brows, use a stick or wand concealer that's slightly lighter than your skintone, suggests make-up artist Trish McEvoy. 'Literally use it to draw down the line, extending the line slightly at either end of the furrow. Then blend by patting with a finger. It creates an optical illusion, making the line less visible.' Yves Saint Laurent's Touche Eclat is a favourite of make-up artists for the same trick.

■ Prescriptives Magic Invisible Line Smoother can be used to 'fill' a frown-line, to make it look less deep. (For more about this truly 'magic' product, see page 77.)

■ JOEY New York (see RESOURCES) have created what they call 'the safe alternative to BOTOX®': a line-filling gel called Line Up that can be used wherever you might have a filler, which has a mild tightening effect. Has to be worth a shot. (Or rather, worth a try before getting that shot...)

■ Devotees of facial exercises believe that they can help combat frown-lines (among other facial flaws). Facial workout guru Eva Fraser (see RESOURCES) suggests the following workout to eliminate horizontal lines on the forehead.

1   Sit in front of a mirror, rest your elbows on a table and place the pads of your fingertips along your hairline.

2   Gently push your brow upwards and hold, keeping your head erect.

3   Looking straight ahead, bring your brow down in five movements against the resistance of your hold and, as you do so, gradually close your eyes.

4   Hold this downward pull for a count of three, then slowly release.

5   Don't scowl or push your head into your hands – it can cause tension in the back of your neck.

6   Remember to relax and breathe.

7   Repeat three times.

CHAPTER 4

Fill 'em up – the injectables

Laughter lines. Smile lines. Wrinkles. Crow's feet. Whatever you call them, these are the visible signs of ageing that women most seem to fret about, the evidence of years spent squinting, frowning, laughing, chewing and smiling, as well as time spent in the sun. (And, of course, gravity.) No wonder, then, that soft tissue 'line-filling' has become huge business, carried out in a booming number of clinics the world over.

These injectables can be used to fill in lines and wrinkles, add fullness to the lips (and cheeks, in some cases), fill in scars, and even plump up sunken areas of the face. Injectables are mostly appropriate for deeper furrows and creases, rather than the finer lines (like 'lipstick lines' around the mouth), for which a resurfacing technique – micro dermabrasion, or laser therapy – may be more appropriate. In reality, many experts today use a 'smorgasbord' approach: a bit of filling here, a bit of 'sandblasting' (as I tend to think of it!) there...

Everyone's case – everyone's face – is different, but what this chapter will tell you is exactly what's involved in each 'filling' technique. Based on your evaluation, your anatomy, your lifestyle – and your goals – the doctor should choose the best treatment option for you. If your doctor and/or clinic suggests a two- or three-way approach to turning back the clock, you should also check out the other procedures elsewhere in this book. Personally I believe it's important to look for someone who has experience with many different types of surgical and non-surgical facial procedures. Doctors aren't going to recommend a procedure that they don't offer – only the ones that they do. The wider the range of treatments on offer, the more options at their disposal – and the more likely you are to end up with the perfect procedure for you.

Be aware, meanwhile, that fillers can't help with sagging, bagging or 'jowls', for which a facelift may be the only solution. (If you really want to take that step and can afford a) the cost and b) the 'downtime'.) Another important point to remember is that many of the most widely used fillers offer only a temporary solution which will require expensive maintenance, should you like the results and be keen to keep them up. The body – sooner (usually) or sometimes later – metabolises the material.

There are some injections – soft facial implants like SoftForm™, and injections like Artecoll® and Evolution – which offer more permanent solutions, but you should proceed with extreme caution here, and only once you're 100 per cent satisfied in the skill of your surgeon, and in his or her aesthetic sense. (I've heard plenty of tales of doctors who are medically brilliant, but whose results are less-than-satisfactory because they're not looking at the whole picture – i.e. the whole face, just at the wrinkle being filled.) It's worth bearing in mind that in the world of cosmeto-dermatology, there are Rembrandts out there – and Francis Bacons…

If a permanent filler goes hard at some stage in the future, or moves, or starts to protrude, it will need surgical extraction – and removing permanent fillers tends to be considerably more painful and complicated than putting them in. (From line to scar…) What happens when your face naturally shifts and changes over the years? Some permanent 'filler' injections, over time, have been known to become visible bumps in later life, as the face's own fat disappears. (From wrinkle to ridge…) Maybe it'll take thirty years – but what would you do then? As Manhattan-based Dr Debra Jaliman says,

'Patients always say, "I want something permanent; I don't want to have to come back." But you wouldn't get the same haircut today that you'd get ten years from now. As we age, our faces change. So if you put in a filler that lasts for ever, and then you have a facelift, you'll end up moving the skin with a filler in it. It just wouldn't look right.'

(Incidentally, a word of caution: a couple of years ago when I looked into permanent fillers, some of the doctors I spoke to were giving rave reviews to one particular filler – which is pretty much made from the same stuff as tents and waterproof clothing. Since then, some of those same doctors tell me, they've stopped working with this filler – because as one cosmeto-dermatologist observes, 'It's difficult to work with, it is hard to touch and it can move – sometimes extruding through the side of the lip.' Which only goes to illustrate just how fickle filler fashion is.)

I believe, in any case, you should think extremely carefully about what you allow to be injected into your body. In the US, there are several fillers in use which use collagen harvested from cadavers – dead bodies. Several other fillers (many of which are used here) are animal-derived – and in the light of Mad Cow Disease, or Bovine Spongiform Encephalopathy (BSE, for short), patients may worry about the risk of infection. When the initial outbreak of BSE happened, it is thought that there may have been a potential risk of infection to patients whose collagen could have been sourced from British cattle, potentially resulting in Creutzfeld-Jacob Disease (which leads to brain degeneration and ultimately death). In reality, there has never been a case of infection from collagen – but you may want to ask yourself whether you want any animal by-product in your system, because of the risk of coming into contact not just with known diseases that can cross the species barrier, but perhaps some that haven't yet come to light. (And of course, animal-derived fillers are definitely off the menu for vegetarians...)

Some permanent fillers, meanwhile, are basically made of a type of plastic – and you have to ask yourself how you feel about having that permanently in your body for the rest of your life – even in small quantities. In light of the widely reported health risks associated with silicone injections (see page 72), it's not unreasonable to wonder whether other fillers might turn out to have less-than-desirable side effects, down the road. (These are all issues you should be thinking about, as you weigh up whether or not to have these procedures. By all means, talk through any anxieties with your doctor – but be aware that he may not have the long-term answers, because in truth, nobody does.)

As you read through this chapter, don't use this section as a 'shopping list', or go to see a surgeon and try to strong-arm him or her into giving you a particular treatment based solely on what you've read here; I'm certainly not here to recommend which filler (if any) is most appropriate to your specific map of lines and wrinkles. An experienced cosmetic surgeon or cosmeto-dermatologist will have his or her preferred techniques and products for filling lines. (Fillers are known in medical circles as 'devices', incidentally – a phrase that refers to the filler itself, not the equipment for introducing it.)

What I recommend is that after you discuss your individual case with each expert you visit for a preliminary consultation, you use this section to do your homework so that you know exactly what's involved (including an account 'from the horse's mouth' of someone who's had it done), and so that you're aware of just what will be put in your body, and what happens to it there. I've seen some women be as casual about going for filler injections as if they were buying a new lipstick, whereas I believe that any cosmeto-dermatological procedure – not just filler injections, but laser resurfacing or micro-dermabrasion – should only be embarked upon if you've really wised up first.

It's important to choose the person who's going to give you your treatment with great care – and not to be rushed. If this is your first time, shop around, compare facilities and 'bedside manner', as well as prices. (Which can vary wildly.) Some syringe-wielders are definitely more qualified than others. Says Dr Carruthers: 'I know of people without any formal training carrying out injections or operating machines while the doctor they work for is on his boat, or in the emergency room.' (The fact that this is illegal doesn't stop it happening.)

As for recovery time? Are these really 'lunchtime' procedures? Be aware that age, genetic background, skin quality and lifestyle – as well as the injected site – may all play a role in how well (and how quickly) you recover; if you bruise badly when you so much as gently knock into a chair, you're more likely to be one of the patients who goes black and blue after a 'filler' injection. If you tend to be resilient to bruising, that will probably indicaye a quick recovery from these procedures. Dr Carruthers points out, meanwhile, that even procedures which are touted as being allergy-free may trigger problems in a few individuals. 'Nothing is ever zero risk of reaction,' he says, 'because even if you're not allergic to the material itself, it's possible to have a reaction to the tiny amounts of other material which are in the injection.'

If you do go ahead, ask your doctor/nurse for a sheet of instructions to follow before and after the procedure, to minimise risks – and do so, to the letter. With every kind of filler, if you experience a local reaction that doesn't resolve itself in a few days, get back in touch with the person who treated you to discuss this.

Artecoll®

(NB Artecoll® is an updated version of the filler formerly known as Arteplast).

The low-down Artecoll® is tiny microspheres of inert PMMA (polymethulmethacrylate) – a form of plastic, basically – suspended in a collagen solution. PMMA has a long history of use – for instance, in hip joint replacement, repair of skull defects, artificial lenses etc. The idea is that after injection, the collagen dissipates – leaving the plastic beads behind to plump the skin. Like some other injections, Artecoll® has a built-in anaesthetic, but first, the area is usually anaesthetised with a topical numbing cream. The filler is best applied using a 'linear threading' technique – i.e., a long injection drawn along the length of the wrinkle, rather than many pin-pricks, which could create a 'string of pearls' effect. During the ninety days following treatment, the collagen – which is animal in origin – disperses through the body; the idea is that production of new collagen is stimulated, to surround the acrylate particles in the Artecoll®. It takes three months to establish the full results – and leave long before you should decide whether or not you're happy with them. More can be added – but it can't be taken away.

Suitable for Artecoll® is most suited to filling deep lines, pumping up the lip silhouette, for 'evening up' the nose – and also for inverted nipples. It may also be used for filling depressions – such as acne scars and sunken areas under the eyes.

Not suitable for Anyone who has an allergy to collagen; before you can have Artecoll® treatment, you must have a collagen test to establish if you react to it. Crow's feet and wrinkles in very thin skin are not suitable candidates for Artecoll®.

Recovery time Most people can return to their routine straight from the surgery – applying make-up after a couple of hours if any of the following occur: swelling, tenderness or redness. (Although these shouldn't last more than a day or two.)

The risks The biggest risk is that the skill of the person you've chosen for your Artecoll® treatment doesn't live up to your expectations, and you don't like the results – because they're very hard to reverse. Persistent lumps and bumps – also known as granuloma – are not unknown. These are balls of hard material which form in reaction to the injection and are usually treated with steroid injection into the affected area. There are also anecdotal reports, when Artecoll® has been used as a 'lip-plumper' in the fleshy part of the lips, of it becoming 'rubbery' after three to five years. According to insiders, meanwhile, the 'serious complication rate' is less than 1 in 10,000. Scarring and serious allergy are described as 'very rare'. But it's got to be someone. According to Dr James D. Romano, one of the doctors involved in the Food and Drink Administration trials of Artecoll® in the US, 'Many doctors impulsively judge this as just another foreign substance similar to silicone and fraught with the same set of potential risks and complications. This is simply not the case.' (See SILICONE, page 72.) Because of the permanence of this 'filler', however, you should be absolutely sure that the person who's injecting you is a fully trained – and highly experienced – dermatologist or cosmetic surgeon, who's used to using Artecoll®. If it goes wrong – or you don't like the results – it's extremely difficult to remove.

Upkeep Artecoll® is permanent – once it's there, it's there (although the original collagen is redistributed in the body after 90 days).

How much it costs Prices vary from £400–£700 per session.

CASE STUDY   **'I had Artecoll® for facial lines'**

– JENNY, 44

'As I've gotten older, I've started to look in the mirror and think, "God, I look tired." I have my own consulting business and I am in the public eye a lot; I keep myself physically very fit but it doesn't matter how well you work out, that face doesn't get the workout with you. The area that bugged me most before I had my treatment was the lower part of my face. I'm pretty lean, and I was looking tired, acquiring deep lines that ran from nose to mouth. I didn't have jowls, because I've always believed in non-surgical facelifts (see page 173), which do a great job at firming the jaw.

'Initially, I tried some BOTOX® – which worked well on my forehead frown-line – and Hylaform. But the Hylaform – which initially looked great – disappeared real fast from my face; it was out of my system in a month to six weeks, which is way too high-maintenance for me. That adds up to a lot of money. (I have no idea if this is connected with the fact that I was continuing my non-surgical facelift treatments, but it strikes me that it might have been.) There was also a mis-communication with my doctor; on early sessions, he'd injected the borders of the lips to enhance them and to "puff out" the feathery lines around my mouth, but the third time, he injected the lip itself and I hated the result. I got home and my husband said to me, "what are you doing to yourself…?" I really began to question that myself, too, but the whole episode served to underline to me how very important it is to make sure that the patient and doctor are speaking the exact same language…

'After discussion with the doctor, we decided to try again with Artecoll®, which gives permanent results. The injections themselves really don't bother me; I feel almost no pain or even discomfort as he injects. It fills right away, but I didn't want it all done in one go; the same lines have been filled over three treatments, building up to the point where I can say, "OK, I'm a hundred per cent happy; we can stop now." It's given me a much more refreshed look – although at the same time, I've had braces and a new haircut, so that nobody can quite put their finger on what it is that I've had done, and I'd rather they didn't know. (Having said that, among my girlfriends, there's a bunch of us getting different stuff done, typically, with careers, who are simply not prepared to age the way our mothers did.)

'The bottom line? Nowadays, even when I'm tired, I don't look so tired – and that's what I was aiming for.'

(For a case history of Artecoll® as a lip-plumper, see page 84.)

Autologous fat injections

The low-down Also known as microlipoinjection, this is a technique in which fat is removed by syringe from a patient's buttocks, abdomen or thighs and is inserted to fill out facial lines, wrinkles and depressions. In the 1990s, autologous fat injections were the biggest beauty buzz after BOTOX®, but now that so many other fillers have reached the market, it's dwindling in popularity. The 'donor' site is first cleansed and anaesthetised before the doctor makes a small incision, from which fat is withdrawn using a 'micro-cannula' (small suction implement), or a large-bore syringe. Before the fat can be reinjected, it may be treated so that blood, anaesthetic and any other material is removed. Doctors use several separation techniques – including a centrifuge (which rapidly spins the extracted liquid), or simply decanting the material and allowing it to 'settle' in a test tube; just like in a salad dressing the fat will separate from the other liquid. A saline solution can also be used to purify the fat cells. The fat cells are then reinjected, sometimes at a future appointment, with a large syringe when the area will be locally anaesthetised and sometimes 'marked' using a Magic Marker (to outline the target for the doctor). The fat is then kneaded into position. (Says Dr Patricia Wexler: 'My strong thumbs are my most valuable asset. I don't ski with poles because I'm afraid of dislocating them!') Unlike collagen, which is injected into the skin's superficial layer, fat is injected under the skin into the body's own fat layer. (Which is why it's no good for finer lines.) As a result, the doctors can use more 'filler'. 'Overfilling' is necessary, to allow for the fat to be absorbed in the weeks after surgery. When fat is used to fill in sunken cheeks, or to correct imperfections other than lines, the newly injected fat can have the effect of making the face look swollen.

Suitable for Deeper lines and wrinkles. Autologous fat injections are also one of the few treatments that can 'plump up' ageing hands, although in reality, very few doctors are doing this. Because it's your own fat, you're not likely to be allergic to it. According to Dr Jean-Louis Sebagh (originally from France, but practising in London's Harley Street), 'Women age in one of two ways – they melt or sag.' This fat technique, as Dr Sebagh explains, fills in dark circles and hollow cheeks and gives volume to women who are 'melters'. Before, there were only facelifts, which produce a tight, flat face without volume. (NB Some people having liposuction opt for fat implants as a 'by-product' of their treatment.)

Not suitable for Those without the flesh to transfer; some women are turned down because they simply don't have enough fat to give.

Recovery time No bandages are required on the face but you may be advised to go without make-up for twenty-four hours – making it difficult (if you rely on make-up as 'camouflage') to go straight back to work, or to socialise. If a large area was treated, you may need to curtail your activity for a few days. There is likely to be bruising or swelling at the 'removal' site, less so at the 'injection' site, but the severity of the reaction depends mostly on the size and location of the treated area; some patients have to wait six weeks for their faces to recovery totally. It is necessary to stay away from the sun while the redness and bruising goes down – and in the meantime, after the first twenty-four hours, to apply make-up with sunblock protection as camouflage for your condition.

The risks Fat isn't always absorbed evenly; some areas take it better than others. However, there may be a risk of infection either at the 'donor' site or at the point at which the fat is injected.

Upkeep Fat injections can last around three months – but some patients 're-absorb' the fat much more quickly, making it a high-maintenance option. Initially, you may require several treatments to get your desired result. With repeated injections, it's been claimed, results may begin to last longer because some of the fat allegedly becomes incorporated into the surrounding tissue, establishing its own blood supply.

How much it costs From approximately £300 up, up, up.

CASE STUDY 'I had fat transferred to my face
– and SoftForm™ for wrinkles'

– LAETITIA, 55

'I hit fifty and thought, "It's time to do something" – and I am not interested in a facelift. I wanted something which meant I could be in and out fast, wasn't surgical and didn't require hospitalisation. (Not least because three years ago, I was diagnosed with breast cancer, and I'd had enough operations, thanks. But at the same time I also thought: "I've got so many goddammed doctors, I want to have a fun doctor, for something positive!")

'I have a friend who'd had disastrous cosmetic laser treatment which left her with scarring. To try to deal with this she was referred to Dr Nicholas Lowe, who not only has a private practice but also works as a professor of dermatology at UCLA. He got rid of her scarring to a remarkable extent using gentler lasers – and I thought, "This guy knows what he's doing", and that he was the man for me.

'I started with BOTOX®, which worked beautifully – it was instant gratification and my face looked better from the next day onwards. (I had bad squint-lines; I'm an architect and I always seem to be losing my spectacles, screwing up my eyes and forehead for close work.) In fact, I don't have much sun damage – I freckle easily and have kept out of the sun – and my skin is quite good. But the first signs of ageing that I'd noticed staring back at me from the mirror were deep nose-to-mouth lines – and believe me, they weren't getting any better. So Dr Lowe recommended fat injections for the lines that run from nose to mouth, using fat harvested from my own body. Since I have no shortage of that, it seemed like a great solution! He told me I could pick the area of my body I wanted the fat harvested from – and it was kind of eeny, meeny, miny, mo; I ended up choosing my stomach because it seemed easiest to access.

'I must say that I was very nervous the first time, not knowing what to expect. For the harvesting procedure, I lay down and had a local anaesthetic in my stomach. Then a tiny cannula (or metal tube) is pushed into the skin, and it pumps a water-like substance with a built-in anaesthetic under the skin, separating the fat from the skin; you can literally feel the pressure of the skin and fat coming apart. It expands everything and you wait about ten minutes for the anaesthetic to kick in. The whole process is uncomfortable but it doesn't hurt. Then the fat is sucked out through the cannula – accompanied by slight gurgling, sucky sounds, which is a bit disconcerting. In the event, the amount of fat that comes out is tiny – about four syringe-fuls, in my case. If you want, you can watch it going into the tube; it's yellow-looking, tinged with pink, which is the blood. The openings themselves were very small, though: one under the belly button, one to each side. The first time I had this done, he put in a stitch; the second time, just a plaster. The fat is then taken away to be processed, and the excess stored in a refrigerator for up to one year; after that, it's past its use-by date and you need to have the mini-liposuction done again. (Although next time, I think I might go for the full liposuction and really get rid of my stomach, too. The amount that comes out for facial injections makes no impact on middle-aged spread whatsoever.)

'For the re-injection, a topical anaesthetic is applied, and then with a needle, a local anaesthetic is injected just under the skin. To me, this is the most painful and uncomfortable part of the whole process, including the mini-liposuction. When you're totally numb, he shoots the fat in through a very fine needle, at several points along the fold.

With a surgically-gloved hand, the doctor then manipulates the fat in the line until it's placed where he's happy with it. Altogether, I counted four points of entry for the needle on one side, three on the other, because the line's not symmetrical. I can see tiny puncture marks – but nobody else would probably notice – and I get a little local redness bruising on my face, because I'm a bruiser; I take a blood-thinning drug for arthritis, which of course I explained during my consultation. Indeed, my stomach goes totally black and blue after the liposuction – but it doesn't trouble me because nobody's going to see it. And frankly, I've had these injections done at 4 p.m. and gone straight out to dinner that night.

'The first fat injections looked great immediately and I was delighted. But the benefits of the fat injections disappeared within a month and a half, and Dr Lowe explained that's just what happens with some people. In others, the fat sticks around longer. I had the injections a couple of times and it was proving very high-maintenance so he recommended that I also have SoftForm™ in the lines, too. Then we could wait and see if I needed fat layered over the top.

'Before he did the SoftForm™, I was again very nervous, so I asked for a Valium – and got one, so that by the time the local anaesthetic was applied, I didn't care about a thing. During the procedure, he first made four small incisions – just in the crease below the nose, where it can barely be seen, and at the other end of the line, near my mouth, on both sides; for this, he uses his aesthetic judgement – and that's why it's so important to go to someone good. Then with a needle he threads the SoftForm™ into the line between the incisions. This requires a lot of pressure; I remember it was uncomfortable and it felt like my face was being somewhat manhandled. The whole thing took about ten to fifteen minutes, after the topical had kicked in – probably about twenty minutes, for that. Immediately after the SoftForm treatment, I looked in a magnifying mirror and could see that the incisions looked absolutely tiny. They were closed with tiny stitches using clear thread, over which Dr Lowe had sprayed a liquid bandage to seal the wound and allow make-up to be applied immediately over the top. This took around four days to peel off (although there was nothing visible to anyone else's naked eye), and then I went back to have the stitches out. I remember being a bit sore and bruised, and shaky – from the sheer physical assault of having someone working closely on my face, which is how I've sometimes felt after the dentist. But I went to dinner and the theatre that night without a qualm. I was warned not to have major dental work for a few weeks, though, so that the filler stays perfectly in place.

'Looking in the mirror, the lines had almost disappeared. If I touched them with my finger, for the first few months, I could sense what felt like a piece of spaghetti running down them – but only if I was actually trying to feel for it; there's no strange sensation otherwise. Then within around five months, my own collagen had wrapped around the SoftForm™ and now I can barely feel a thing if I touch it.

'I now have fat injections every three to four months over the SoftForm™, and the results are wonderful; I'm very, very pleased. I might have had this done sooner if I'd known it existed. I don't go around advertising what I've had done but friends can see the difference. They think I've had a new haircut, or something. And that's just fine.'

Collagen Replacement Therapy®
(aka Zyderm®/Zyplast®)

The low-down Collagen protein is the main component of the dermis, or deep layer of skin, and gives skin its natural suppleness; as the years roll by, natural collagen is lost – leading to facial lines and wrinkles. (NB Although some skin creams contain collagen, this ingredient – when formulated into a cream – is only there for its moisturising/emollient properties and cannot replace the skin's own lost collagen.) The idea with collagen injections is to use an animal-derived version (from calf's skin and/or hooves) to top up the skin's own dwindling supply. Although there is an anaesthetic agent (lidocaine) mixed in with the collagen, a local anesthetic may be used if you are particularly sensitive to pain – a topical cream anaesthetic or a numbing spray. Collagen is then injected by the dermatologist/ aesthetician in several spots along the line to 'fill' it and puff it up, using an ultra-fine needle only slightly thicker than a human hair. The effects are immediate: lines are greatly diminished. However, since part of the substance is salt water that will be absorbed by the body within a few days, the doctor will slightly overfill the area – so the initial impression can be misleading. You may be asked to hold a hand mirror during the procedure to help the doctor decide when you've had enough. The procedure takes approximately ten minutes per line but can vary from patient to patient and, of course, on length of line.

Suitable for The feathery lines around lips, frown lines, crow's feet; it's said to be particularly good for the lines running from nostrils to the corners of the mouth. Also used for lip-plumping (to create the famous 'Paris pout') and for filling acne scars. Your doctor will decide whether Zyderm I® or Zyderm II® (which smooth finer lines and wrinkles) or Zyplast® (which is suitable for deeper creases and furrows), or a combination of these, is most appropriate for you.

Not suitable for Collagen is contra-indicated for people with arthritis, lupus or immuno-deficiencies; some people – around 3 per cent, it's thought – are allergic to collagen and to establish this, a test is carried out around a month before actual treatment, using a test site (usually the forearm). In minor cases of allergy, skin turns red, itches and peels; in more serious cases, it can turn red and start flaking and oozing; any symptoms at all at the 'test site' should be reported to your doctor. Collagen is also off-limits for pregnant women and anyone who's allergic to beef or beef products, as well as to lidocaine (the anaesthetic agent that's contained in the syringe along with the collagen).

Recovery time Immediately after treatment, you may experience minor discomfort, throbbing or stinging in the injected area; in some patients there's bruising, swelling and/or small bumps – but this is usually minor. Any redness tends to disappear within twenty-four hours – although in fair patients, this redness can be obvious for up to a week. Tiny scabs may also form over the needle-entry areas, but you can apply make-up directly after treatment to disguise any problems.

The risks Collagen has been used in different medical applications for over a hundred years – including for stitches and replacing faulty heart valves. However, because some people are allergic to collagen – in extreme cases, this can lead to shock and difficulty breathing and/or muscle pain – patients must be tested for sensitivity first. Those allergic aren't suitable candidates for this particular 'filler' injection; cases of delayed allergy aren't unknown, ranging from hives to breathing problems. (These may then treated with steroids.) People with specific diseases may be more at risk of allergy than others – for instance, rheumatoid arthritis (and the juvenile form of this illness), and scleroderma. Other risks not necessarily linked with allergies include infection, abscesses, open sores, skin peeling, scars and lumpiness, which may persist over the treated area; some patients have apparently reported small red dots sprouting along wrinkle lines where shots were given, taking a year or two to disappear. (Although it should be pointed out that reports of these problems are extremely rare.) There's also a controversy over whether bovine collagen might cause auto-immune diseases (such as lupus, dermatomyositis and polymyositis) – in which the body mistakenly starts attacking its own cells – although this hasn't been proved. Although the notoriously cautious Food and Drink Administration in the US has approved collagen for filling in 'contour deformities' in the skin (such as scars and wrinkles), it hasn't been approved for lip-plumping. The FDA themselves point out: 'Because collagen stays in the body and continues to be absorbed, the possible effects of collagen injections before or during pregnancy are unknown.'

Upkeep Collagen is gradually re-absorbed into the body and top-ups need to be done every six months, minimum – more likely every three to four; on lips the effect is more short-lived, wearing off in (usually) six to eight weeks.

How much it costs Approximately £350 per syringe; people with very deep or numerous lines may need two to three syringes at one go.

(NB Coming down the line: a new collagen, produced from the donated foreskin of healthy newborn boy, which is expected to cause few, if any, allergic reactions, called CosmoDerm 1 NST – short for No Skin Testing. Nice!)

CASE STUDY   **'I had collagen for facial lines'**

– ANNA, 50

'I've had collagen three to four times a year for the last five years – and frankly, I dont mind admitting that I'm addicted. I'm now fifty, but I don't think anyone would say I looked it. I have it done purely for myself – vanity; I'm just not going to grow old gracefully. I've never been in the sun, so I have it done to reverse the effects of natural ageing. The areas where I have the collagen are in the lines from nose to mouth, and on top of the lip. Originally I'd been considering a full facelift, but at forty-five, the clinic I went to see talked me out of it – and asked if I'd heard of collagen, instead. (I hadn't.)

'The first time, I was absolutely petrified, but the nurse applied some numbing cream (local anaesthetic) and I didn't feel a thing. When the cream had taken effect, she wiped it off and I was asked to sit down on a couch in a cubicle, given a mirror and told to lean forward so that the lines showed up. We then agreed which lines needed to be filled. She took the needle and attached it to a vial of collagen; then I lay back, listening to relaxing music, and she filled the lines discussed, using tiny pin-pricks. I couldn't feel a thing, except a bit of pressure when she put a rubber-gloved finger inside my mouth as if "squashing" the line from the inside (as well as the outside) – to disperse the collagen into the line. When each line was done, I'd lean forward and look in the mirror again to check the progress.

'Now, for my top-ups, when I arrive at the clinic, I'm given the cream and told to rub it in myself while I wait for my appointment. I put it all over the surrounding area – from the nose to the top of the mouth, and around the whole area to be treated. I'll be sitting there in the waiting area with other patients – and we're all slathered in this cream. It's about as glamorous as having highlights done with foils in the hairdresser, but actually, it's quite a bonding experience as we all sit there chatting!

'If I'm feeling flush with money and I see a line, I'll go after six weeks and have half a vial of collagen – a purely selfish one. Or if I'm not feeling so well-off, I'll go for my regular treatment and tell her I can only afford one-and-a-half vials. Overall, treatment usually takes about twenty to twenty-five minutes and I never get a sense of being rushed. She makes sure that if it's lunchtime, I look fine to go back to work – and always asks if I want some make-up on afterwards. (Usually I don't; on me, there's no redness, no mark.) It can take up to an hour before the local anaesthetic wears off, though – so you can't eat or drink anything without risking making a fool of yourself.

'I can't think of a downside. I'm hooked and I love it and I don't look fifty – and that's because of collagen. I factor it into my whole overall annual "grooming" costs: hair, nails, tint, collagen. Now I've no idea what I look like without the collagen – and I have no intention of ever finding out.'

(For a case history of collagen as a lip-filler, see page 86)

DermaLive®

(NB This is available in a version for more prominent furrows and wrinkles, called DermaDeep.)

The low-down No allergy test is required for DermaLive®, which is made up of hyaluronic acid and acrylic hydrogel particles (a type of plastic, if you like); acrylic hydrogel has been used in cataract surgery for some years. It's called a 'hydrogel' because actually, the material has a high water content (25%). The idea is that the hyaluronic acid is metabolised by the body, allowing the acrylic hydrogel to be distributed in the dermis (deeper in the skin), just where it's needed. Over time, these particles are surrounded by the body's own collagen, which completes the 'fill' of the area. A fine needle is used; the DermaLive® is injected into the line as the needle is drawn out – and the procedure takes around ten to fifteen minutes.

Suitable for Medium and deep wrinkles, frown lines, laughter lines, lines around the mouth, nose-to-lip creases and acne scars.

Not suitable for Fine lines.

Recovery time Redness and swelling, with or without pain, can develop after the injection but usually calms down of its own accord after a few days.

The risks Very rarely, localised inflammation can flare up several months after the injection; the whole area becomes hard, sometimes with swelling and redness. This may be treated with steroid creams.

Upkeep DermaLive® is said (by some practitioners) to deliver longer-lasting results than many fillers. Of the initial 'fill', around 40 per cent is retained in the dermis – and overall, the results are claimed to last several years. According to the company's information, DermaLive® 'has been used in France for three years with the effects still visible'. Two or three treatments are usually required, initially, for optimum benefits.

How much it costs From £400 per syringe.

CASE STUDY   'I had DermaLive® for nose-to-mouth lines and chin enhancement'

– PETER, 36

'I work in IT recruitment in a very "laddish" environment where appearances nevertheless matter a lot. I've gotten very into male grooming in the last few years, I go to the gym three or four times a week, get my hair cut regularly – and so having filler injections was really a logical step on from that. I felt there was a little more that I could do to look good, and that a bit now was better than a lot later. If you're fifty and sagging like hell, then you're going to need to go in for all kinds of nips and tucks...

'Initially, I had hair transplants, and I was shopping around for other treatments that might be suitable. I have an Italian look to me, generally good skin – something people comment on – but I was a bit concerned that my lines stood out a bit, especially those running from nose to mouth; my girlfriend commented on them, too. I had an all-in-one consultation followed immediately by treatment. I was initially quite wary and sceptical but I found the environment very comfortable – like a beautiful flat, rather than a surgery, and that felt quite reassuring and relaxed. It seemed to take away any of the stigma attached to what I was doing.

'Compared to the hair transplant – in which even the local anaesthetic was absolute agony – this was a breeze; just a little bit of pain, enough to make my eyes water but nothing worse than that. (There was no pre-injection anaesthetic.) For the nose to mouth, the needle was inserted along the line itself and then drawn out again. I also had what's called "chin enhancement", in which my chin was slightly built up with several injections.

'I had redness for about two or three hours – it looked like razor burn; just a minor irritation and certainly nothing serious. Of course, I was looking in the mirror every ten minutes to see some kind of improvement, but it really only became obvious the next day: the lines were less depressed and obvious, and I'd say I looked younger. I went away for that weekend and got a bit of sun and when I came back on the Monday, people really did say to me, "You look radiant!"

'I feel because I've started having this done while I'm quite young, I've got pretty good results. Obviously if you have the haggard face of a mountain climber, you're not going to get the same effect, but I'm delighted and plan to have it done twice a year, for maintenance. I wouldn't hesitate to have something else done, now, if I felt I needed it. The DermaLive® has caused a little bit of friction with my girlfriend, though; she says "What did you need to go and have that done for?" – but to be honest, she was the same about my hair transplant. As far as I'm concerned, it's about feeling better in yourself – and I do. She's probably just jealous.'

Evolution

The low-down Evolution is a permanent filler. It's made up of microscopic, Malteser-like particles of polyvinyl, suspended in a viscoelastic polyacrylamide gel. The word 'viscoelastic' is quite key: it means that it flows freely within the skin, making it easy for the person injecting it to reach the precise target. What makes Evolution different from other permanent fillers, is that previously, implants have worked by a process called 'accretion' – inducing a foreign-body reaction, as the body tries to deal with the implant. (Something that's neither controllable or predictable.) Once Evolution is injected, this implant apparently has a positive electrical charge, which attracts negatively charged molecules towards it – notably 'good guys' like hyaluronic acid, collagen and elastin – and ultimately creating a stable, 3D network in the skin; the process stops, naturally, when a balance has been reached. The boost in hyaluronic acid makes the skin springier, and creates a sponginess around the implant that gives a natural feel. The gel itself, meanwhile, then takes around two to three years to degrade in the body, leaving the spheres in place, which have become part of the body's own tissues. 'The end result is little polyvinyl spheres embedded in your natural collagen mesh,' explains Dr Elisabeth Dancey, who's been pioneering its use as a filler in the UK. No initial allergy test is required, because Evolution (and Outline, it's near relation) do not contain any known allergenic materials.

Suitable for Deeper lines and wrinkles – such as nose-to-mouth lines, chin lines, forehead lines – folds, scars and areas in and below the skin where tissue has been lost. It can also be used for enhancing mouth volume, and is sometimes used in tandem with its sister product, Outline (see page 66), which has a shorter 'body life' – of two years.

Not suitable for Anyone who's nervous about the possible long-term effects of leaving any man-made substance in the body for years and years, merely for cosmetic benefits.

Recovery time Initially, there may be slight swelling – which should be easily disguised with make-up. Once this subsides, the line will retain around 65 per cent of the original volume of the filler.

The risks If for whatever reason you don't like the results, you're stuck with them; because the filler is surrounded by the body's own tissues, it could theoretically be removed – but probably not without scarring.

Upkeep Normally a single treatment is enough, but this can be repeated four to six weeks later, for further filling. Because Evolution is permanent, you should not need a 'top-up' in future – but it's human biology for lines and creases to continue to deepen, so they won't be erased for ever with this treatment.

How much it costs Prices may vary from £250 to £400 per treatment.

CASE STUDY   'I had Evolution'

– ELIZABETH, 35

'I work in investment banking which is about as lookist and youth-orientated a world as it's possible to be in. I felt I was developing lines running from my nose to my mouth, and I wanted to erase them. A pure vanity thing. From a professional perspective, the younger and more attractive you look, the more business you get. End of story. I had my Evolution from Dr Elisabeth Dancey, who I see for BOTOX®, and who told me that this was a deeper, permanent filler that would be suitable for these grooves. (I love the BOTOX®. I'm addicted. What's also amazing, to me, is that since I've been having it done, I haven't suffered from migraines, which have blighted me all my adult life.)

'She rubbed in some EMLA (numbing) cream, and after ten minutes I couldn't feel a thing. It's a deep injection, right into the lines, and although I wasn't particularly red afterwards, within twelve hours I'd bruised like hell – probably because the jab is so deep. I am not really someone who bruises, so this was a surprise – although I hadn't taken any arnica, which I think might have helped prevent the bruising. To be honest, the bruises lasted for weeks and during the purple stage they were really hard to camouflage; less so when the bruise became a green-y/yellow. But the bottom line is that I only had to have this done once, so the trade-off was worth it.

'Initially, the line was a little fuller, then it deflated after a couple of weeks, and then filled out again – as the body's own collagen production kicked in. (I don't think anyone else would have noticed this inflating and deflating, though; it's quite subtle.)

'I have a lot of girlfriends who think this kind of thing is appalling, and would never do it. Somehow it's fine to have your hair done and even your teeth fixed, but to mess around with your face is somehow not done. To me, all this is like buying nice clothes – less than half the cost of buying a new upmarket designer suit, and it will hopefully last a lot longer. So what the hell?'

Hylaform

The low-down Hylaform Viscoelastic Gel (to give it its full name) is touted as a 'low allergy' filler because it doesn't require a skin test – unlike collagen. (But it's still not suitable for everyone – see below.) In fact, Hylaform is a derivative of a joint-lubrication material, hyaluronic acid, which is found in human and animal tissue (and is also an ingredient in some skin creams where it acts as an effective moisturiser). The area is first treated with a topical anaesthetic, and the filler injected at intervals just under the skin's surface through a very fine needle. Once in place, the Hylaform is massaged by the doctor to smooth the material.

Suitable for Lines across the forehead and between the brows (frown-lines) – although BOTOX® is the No. 1 treatment-of-choice here – as well as nose-to-mouth lines, smoker's lines, crow's feet, acne scars and lip-plumping. Hylaform can be used on patients who have had a positive skin test for collagen.

Not suitable for Finer lines and wrinkles. Anyone who has an allergy to chicken or eggs is not a candidate for Hylaform, though, as the key ingredient comes from rooster combs.

Recovery time As with most filler injections, there may be swelling and redness for between twenty-four to forty-eight hours, which you should be able to cover with make-up; a small percentage of patients experience signs of skin irritation, including itching.

The risks According to Dr Ellen Gendler, who's been involved in the testing of Hylaform in the US, 'In my own experience, placement of the material too superficially results in surface bumps, while injection too deep produces a very short-lived effect that perhaps lasts for only one day.' Doctors, she pointed out, must establish for themselves 'how it is best delivered'. (So to avoid being a guinea pig you want to establish that the person injecting you has done this hundreds of times.)

Upkeep According to Dr Nicholas Lowe, Clinical Professor of Dermatology at UCLA School of Medicine with offices just off Harley Street and in Santa Monica, Hylaform is longer-lasting than some implants – but certainly not as permanent as many patients would wish; three months onwards seems to be the consensus. (It may be – as with other fillers – that in some patients, the hyaluronic gel is absorbed and metabolised more quickly than in other patients.) Long-term human studies are still being carried out on how well Hylaform 'goes the distance'; in animal studies, the implants were still perceptible at six months – but not after one year.

How much it costs Prices vary from £170 to £300.

CASE STUDY   'I have regular Hylaform treatments'

― Carla, 42

'I've been having filler injections since I first noticed a few smile lines around my eyes – and a deepening of the line from nose-to-mouth – when I was in my early 30s, so that's nearly a decade now. When I stopped smiling, I could see that my lines were still there – and I didn't like it; my background is in modelling and I suppose I'm very conscious of what I look like.

'Since then, I've been having Collagen Replacement Therapy® and Hylaform – sometimes one, sometimes the other. I simply can't imagine not having them, now. The two techniques are very similar, although with collagen, there's an anaesthetic in the injection itself, so the area doesn't have to be pre-numbed, as it does with Hylaform. This is done with an EMLA cream, which takes about 20 minutes to have an effect before my doctor injects the Hylaform in a series of small pin-prick injections. However, even with the numbing cream, I still find this really quite painful – on a scale of one to ten, I'd say it scored seven in the pain stakes – compared to four for collagen.

'Immediately after the injection, the area is also a bit bumpy; this slight lumpiness -under the surface of the skin along the line at the points of entry – lasts for about a week or two weeks. It definitely bothers me – although it probably isn't noticeable to anyone else – but isn't bad enough to stop me going to work or out to dinner. For me, despite this (and the pain factor), the advantage of Hylaform over collagen is that it lasts just that little bit longer – three months, as opposed to two for collagen, which can be an issue in a busy life. It also seems to fade less slowly – it's not a gradual dwindling; I just wake up one morning after about three months, look at my lines and think: "OK, it's time for a top-up". I'm always pleased with the results with both fillers, but on balance – because there's less pain and no lumpiness – I prefer collagen. If it wasn't for the fact it didn't last as long, I'd always choose that one.

'I will go on having fillers until I feel the need for surgery, and if something better comes along, I might try that, instead. For someone with good, young skin – say up to the age of fifty – these filler injections may be the answer, but they're no substitute for a facelift. Only an operation can remove sags and jowls, and when I look in the mirror and feel the fillers aren't enough any more – I'll be booking in with a surgeon.

NEW-FILL®

Suitable for Fine lines, wrinkles, furrows and creases, and to enhance cheeks, fill baggy rings around the eyes, chin and lips. In addition NEW-FILL® is also being used to 'plump up' scrawny hands and for the saggy skin above the bust-line – and even 'adding volume' to knees on which gravity has taken its toll! Because it's non-animal based (unlike collagen), no patch-testing is needed in advance of treatment.

Not suitable for Like most injections, NEW-FILL® is unsuitable for people with bleeding disorders.

The low-down NEW-FILL® is made up of polylactic acid (which has been used for many years for internal stitching and bone surgery), which is a synthetic polymer. According to the manufacturers, NEW-FILL® has a dual mechanism: as well as the gel filling the wrinkle, it gets to work over time by actually stimulating the skin's own collagen production process, so although there's immediate 'plumping', full results are seen after around twenty days as the collagen-stimulating elements start to work. During the treatment, lines are filled using a fine-gauge needle which makes a long, tunnelling injection into the line, creating the space for the filler, which is deposited as the needle is drawn out; most lines require at least two injections. Although the pain is described generally as 'a little discomfort', anyone with even a whisper of wimpiness is advised to insist on a local anaesthetic gel. Massage may be required in areas like frown-lines to ensure even distribution of the filler.

Recovery time There may be some swelling or redness and/or bruising, but these reactions are described as 'mild' and 'temporary'. Don't be surprised to discover that after two or three days, the initial effect is slightly diminished; the manufacturers insist that it takes almost three weeks to perceive the full improvement.

The risks The technique is extremely precise: too deep an injection will introduce the NEW-FILL® at a deeper level than required to 'fill' the wrinkle – so there are no visible results.

Upkeep Initial treatment calls for two sessions, roughly two to three weeks apart; a third treatment may be required in some patients (particularly if you're over sixty). Most patients should expect a sustained improvement for about a year – or in some cases, longer.

How much it costs From approximately £200.

CASE STUDY

'I had NEW-FILL® for my nose-to-mouth wrinkles'

– NIKKI, 48

'I had breast cancer five years ago, which recurred last year and required radiotherapy, and ever since then I've had this mission that people only have one life and you should look and feel your best for it. I would look in the mirror and although I don't really have sun damage, I literally hated seeing the indentations that ran from my nose to my lips; I felt it was incredibly ageing. I was very impressed at the results on a couple of friends who'd had NEW-FILL®. Then about three months ago I was at a health club for a massage, where I saw someone go in to see the visiting doctor for the treatment – and then saw them again, as they walked out; I just said, "Right, book me in." My husband was very doubtful – he said, "You don't need that, especially after what you've been through." I'm not going to say that I wasn't worried or nervous – and unsure about the idea of having "an alien substance" in my body, after my health troubles – but on balance I decided it was worth going for.

'I had an initial consultation when I was told I'd need two sessions; during the first, they'd use around 75 per cent of the total filler, then a top-up of around 25 per cent. When I actually had it done, the doctor applied the anaesthetic cream – which took around fifteen minutes to kick in – and then I felt a pin-prick, nothing more, as the needle went in. In all, she inserted the needle four times, evenly placed each side along the line, and at the end of the first line placed one gloved finger inside my mouth, one outside, and massaged the line to distribute the filler. She then gave me a mirror to look in after she'd done one side and I knew immediately I was an addict. In all it took no more than five minutes, and I really experienced no pain at all.

'The area around the lines was a little inflamed and puffy immediately afterwards so I applied some make-up before I went home; at that point, it didn't really feel like "me" if I touched the line, but that might have been the anaesthetic. I had the NEW-FILL® around 1 p.m. and by that night, the swelling had subsided enough for me to go out. I am prepared to invest in how I look; I've bought expensive face creams like Crème de la Mer, but this is incomparably better than any cream. A friend asked my husband whether he was against it, and he said, "She looks fantastic, and if it makes her happy, I'm all for it." To be honest, I feel so much better about myself since I've had the filler, I would go so far as to say it's actually helped my recovery from my illness. Certainly, people now comment on how well I look. It's the best thing I could have done. If a woman can look better, why not?'

Outline

The low–down   Like Evolution (see page 58), Outline is a polyacrylamide copolymer – basically, a non-animal, plastic-type gel – but in this case, without the microspheres. According to Dr Dancey,

'It's the same stuff that's in your bra!' Outline was developed by a French research scientist, searching for new, long-lasting materials for use in heart surgery – and of non-animal origin, because of recent scares about possible risk of cross-infection. 'Because the body doesn't know how to deal with the filler,' Dr Dancey continues, 'it basically leaves it where it is – which is why Outline is such a long-lasting filler compared to animal-derived versions, which tend to be rapidly metabolised. It gradually breaks down into non-allergenic particles or fragments within the body.' Used in exactly the same way as Evolution, it is injected into fine lines and wrinkles, as well as deeper lines where the patient doesn't want permanent results.

Suitable for All kinds of deep and fine lines and wrinkles, except those in the eye zone; it can also be used for lip enhancement, where, according to Dr Dancey, it gives exceptional results because 'it's like an implant in a syringe'. Outline can also replace lost volume in cheeks and scar tissue. Because Outline is non-allergenic, it's suitable for patients who react to collagen.

Not suitable for Eye zone – see above.

Recovery time You may be left with a small amount of redness or swelling at the site of the injection which should disappear within twenty-four hours.

The risks See Evolution, page 59.

Upkeep You can expect Outline to last for up to two years before it needs to be re-injected.

How much it costs From approximately £300 per syringe, which should treat more than one line.

'I had Outline'

– LISA, 38

'I have regular Face Magic treatments (see page 181), which I think are amazing. (Although they hurt like hell – sometimes I'm jumping off the bed with the pain, but the pay-off is that it really does stimulate the muscles in my face and make me look fresher and younger; I have these fairly erratically but the benefits seem to last.) Nonetheless, I had some fine, feathery lines around my mouth that were starting to bug me. At the same time, I felt that my lip was getting thinner. Outline seemed like a good solution: not too high-maintenance – it's supposed to last for two years – but I liked the idea that it wouldn't hang around in the body for ever and ever and ever...

'I'd had collagen in the past and it really didn't work for me. For about a week I looked like a twit – I had it in my lips and the results were completely unrealistic, and then the whole thing had disappeared within a month. But then a great girlfriend of mine had Outline and I really liked what it did, filling in her lines. I had a dental injection so that I couldn't feel a thing, and the doctor injected first the fine lines around my mouth and then the lips themselves, just a bit, to "puff them up" a bit. This is a real lunchtime fix; I didn't swell up or bruise – although I took arnica, which may have helped.

'The lines have diminished and although the volume of my lips has probably gone down about 30 per cent since the treatment – which I was told to expect – I really like the effect. I generally feel I don't have to wear so much make-up; the effects are subtle but definitely "there". I like the idea that it ultimately disappears, rather than having some strange foreign substance in your body. I also like the fact that a single injection should last two years – although it's too soon to tell whether that will entirely live up to its promises. In the case of some fillers, which need to keep being redone, I don't think it can be good to keep inflating and deflating the skin, can it? And the way this industry's moving, probably by the time I do go back for a top-up, they'll have something even better.'

Restylane®

(Also available in a form called Perlane® for deeper wrinkles and Restylane Fine Lines® for – yes – fine lines.)

The low–down Restylane is a bio-engineered gel form of hyaluronic acid – it's usually derived as a by-product through the growth of bacteria. Its use is claimed – by the manufacturers – to stimulate the body's own production of hyaluronic acid. Hyaluronic acid is naturally present in the body – although production slows down as we age. Explains leading US cosmeto-dermatologist Dr Fredric Brandt, 'If you think of a bowl of Jell-O with blueberries – our cells – in it, hyaluronic acid is the Jell-O.' (NB Many anti-ageing moisturisers contain hyaluronic acid, but alas, this can't bind with the skin or top up our own supplies – it's there because it's useful as a moisturising ingredient.) Some patients tolerate Restylane® injections without anaesthetic, but this is readily available in the form of ointment or injection – and you should certainly not feel shy of speaking out if it starts to hurt. Treatment takes about ten to fifteen minutes – a series of small injections along the line – and results will be obvious (if a little exaggerated, see below) immediately afterwards.

Suitable for Plumping up wrinkles (it's particularly effective on the lines from nose to mouth) and lip enhancement.

Not suitable for Either very deep or very superficial wrinkles; there are variations-on-a-theme used for this – Restylane Fine Lines® for correcting thin, superficial lines, i.e. around eyes and mouth, including smile lines, while Perlane® – from the same company – is used for enhancing facial contours (for instance, cheeks and chin) or for lip enhancement when additional volume is wanted.

Recovery time In many cases, the treated area swells up and remains red for around twenty-four hours; lips may be swollen and look somewhat uneven for a few days – even up to a week. (I have one friend who had this treatment and has been known, ever since, as 'Donald Duck' by her partner because of the extreme swelling reaction she suffered.)

The risks Up to one in 2,000 people has a quite serious reaction to Restylane® resulting in swelling, redness and tenderness at/near the treatment site, enduring for several weeks after treatment. (Most people, though, are 'able to socialise immediately after treatment'. Though best to steer clear of that glass of champagne till the anaesthetic's worn off, of course.) There are some reports of bumps and 'bubbles' under the skin. One doctor told me that has become wary of using it on patients with very fine, translucent complexions because 'it can be seen, faintly, through the skin'.

Upkeep According to a survey carried out by the manufacturers, after a year, 57 per cent of patients were satisfied with the way Restylane® had worked for them. For the majority of patients, about 50–80 per cent of the effect is still perceptible after six months; most people choose to have treatment re-done after six months – which is certainly the timescale needed to maintain lip contour.

How much it costs Prices may vary from £200+ for Restylane® and approximately £300 for Perlane® per treatment.

CASE STUDY   **'I had Restylane®'**

– SARA, 52

'I am very high-maintenance. I have an appointment with my dermatologist, Dr Fredric Brandt, every single month and he tells me what he thinks I need – sometimes a little BOTOX®, sometimes a peel. I trust him implicitly and if he told me stand on my head for five hours a day I'd do it. If I needed a facelift, I wouldn't hesitate – but what I'm having now, I hope, will keep that day at bay. I don't work – I live off family investments – but I have a busy social life and my appearance is all-important to me. I'm a pretty vain person; I've had my teeth fixed, my ears fixed (because wearing too many earrings as a child stretched the lobes) and I had cosmetic surgery to neaten them up.

'To me, BOTOX® is a miracle for the frown-line on my forehead. But I'd also been having collagen injections for the deep nose-to-mouth lines and I found the collagen disappeared really quickly – in less than three weeks, usually. I read about Restylane® being used in Europe and I used to nag Dr Brandt about it. I was one of the first private patients he treated when he started using it.

'I have an anaesthetic cream applied (which wasn't the case with the collagen injections), and while I lie in a semi-reclining position in the chair, Dr Brandt injects the lines either side of my mouth with the Restylane®. Each line gets about five or six small injections – and I can't feel a thing. (I have friends who've experienced some pain – but not me.)

'There's virtually no swelling, but about twenty-four hours later I do suffer a little bruising at the site of some of the injections – nothing to interfere with my social life, and cover-up cream disguises it. The bruising lasts a week, maximum, and improves every day. What I like about Restylane® is that it lasts much longer than collagen – between four to six months, in my case. If I was neurotic, I'd probably want it every four months, like clockwork. I don't worry about having an "alien substance" in my body – although not everyone I know is so laid-back about it. My sister says to me: "One day you're going to get cancer because of all that stuff you do to yourself," but I've taken a decision: I want to look good, and that's the end of it. What I do believe, though, is that it's vital to find the best doctor you can afford. I have friends who've had bad BOTOX® and bad collagen and the results are awful.

'I may be high-maintenance, but it pays dividends: nobody believes my age. I get loads of compliments; I had my son's room decorated just recently and the painter asked me which kindergarten he was in. He nearly fell off his ladder when I told him my son was thirty-two and working in New York...'

Perlane – See Restylane®, page 69.

Silicone

The low-down Silicone was actually one of the first 'fillers', popularised in the 1960s and 1970s. Microdroplets of medical-grade silicone are injected one-by-one via tiny injections into the lines to be filled, after the area has been locally numbed. However, the whole area of liquid silicone injections is hugely controversial. Several dermatologists I spoke to said that in terms of results, it was a near-perfect choice: long-lasting, versatile, easy-to-use – and if it didn't carry risks, they'd love to use it. But there are very real anxieties about it. (In the US, the FDA has not approved the use of liquid silicone for any cosmetic purposes, including the treatment of facial wrinkles or defects. It is approved for ophthalmic use, i.e. for some eye problems – as a product called AdatoSil – but when it comes to fillers, its use is what's called 'off-label'. In the UK, it's not approved – but that doesn't mean it's not available.)

Suitable for Silicone is used to fill many different depths of line and can also be used to 'plump up' areas such as cheeks and lips. However, there are many, many health question marks over the use of silicone. With the wide range of other options in the beauty world right now, you would be well-advised to think twice – make that two hundred times – before opting for silicone. Nevertheless, silicone still has many advocates among those who used it before the US Food and Drug Administration withdrew appeal – notably Dr Norman

Orentreich, a leading Manhattan-based dermatologist, who's been quite outspoken in its favour – calling it 'the gold standard of filler injections'.

Not suitable for Absolutely anyone who worries about the long-term effects of having this substance floating around in their body. (For floating around, alas, is what can happen...)

Recovery time Short-term, very quick. But long-term? Read on...

The risks According to the FDA themselves, 'The adverse effects of liquid silicone injections have included movement of the silicone to other parts of the body, inflammation and discoloration of surrounding tissues, and the formulation of granulomas – nodules of granulated, inflamed tissue.' There is also a risk of late infection, or of the body rejecting the silicone – pushing the tiny beads through the skin's surface. As a result, a doctor can't legally advertise or sell silicone injections – but it doesn't stop them offering them more discreetly. The use of silicone in breast implants has famously resulted in more serious side effects such as blood clots on the lungs, cancer and even death; there is an entire website of personal horror stories that I stumbled across while surfing the Internet recently. When publicity about this blew up, it prompted a stampede to the doctors' surgeries of women desperate to have their implants removed. Meanwhile, in areas of the US, such as South Florida, there has recently been a flurry of patients getting injected at 'silicone parties' – which is considered a worrying trend by silicone's opponents in the dermatology world.

Upkeep Once it's there, it's there. That's the problem. Removing silicone from, say, a wrinkle, would entail cutting the length of the wrinkle and attempting to remove the material – resulting in a scar. Wrinkle or scar: know which one I'd prefer?

What it costs Silicone injections, where offered, are surprisingly affordable – perhaps because they have to be, to encourage uptake.

I have not included a case history for liquid silicone in this book because of all the 'fillers' I have researched, this is the one that – for now – seems to carry the highest level of serious risk.

SoftForm™

The low-down (Made of a biocompatible polymer called ePTFE) The implant – like a tiny tube – is threaded into skin through tiny cuts and placed underneath the skin behind the lines, creases or wrinkles. (For the mouth, this is usually at the edge of the lips and again in the centre – or the 'peak' of the cupid's bow). The skin is pulled taut and the implant is loaded onto a large, needle-like surgical device called a 'trocar', which is tunnelled into the skin. The ends – which protrude from the puncture holes – are snipped off flush to the skin, and the skin pulled taut to make the ends disappear. (Think of the way you can lose a drawstring in the slits of an elastic waistband...) A small stitch is used to close the incision. The SoftForm™ forms a 'cushion' to lift and support the skin, smoothing the surface so lines are less visible. According to Dr Patricia Wexler, 'skin grows through the length of the tube and surrounds the SoftForm™, so the implant stays put. At the same time, it's Teflon-like – non-stick – so skin doesn't become glued to the implant. If you needed to remove it, you could do so without having to cut out any surrounding skin.' (Not everyone agrees with Dr Wexler's 'non-stick' observation: according to the Facial Plastic Surgery Network, 'Because the SoftForm™ implant is hollow, it allows your tissues to "grow into" the implant. This can make it difficult to remove in the event of an infection.' Observes Dr Fredric Brandt: 'The longer it's in, the harder it is to get out.')

Suitable for Deep creases, furrows – particularly from nose-to-mouth – and flat lip borders; SoftForm™ is increasingly popular as a lip-plumper (see page 83).

Not suitable for Fine lines and wrinkles, acne scars etc.

Recovery time Varies from patient to patient; you may certainly want to duck out of view till the small stitches are removed (although one patient I spoke to simply applied lipstick over the top and went for an audition the next day). There may be residual swelling and soreness, and some patients find it hard to 'pucker up' initially. One woman I spoke to, who had SoftForm™ for both lips and nasolabial folds, said 'I looked like I'd walked into a wall – and although it wasn't impossible to hide with make-up, I'd have taken three or four days off work if I'd known.' Even the official literature for SoftForm™ says: 'Some people have a little bruising or swelling for up to a week; they might need to take a day or two off work.'

The risks As the face becomes thinner, over time, it's possible that the SoftForm™ could start to protrude, in a visibly raised line. Some patients who had the earlier form of SoftForm™ (these implants tend constantly to be 'tweaked' by the manufacturers) complain that they can feel it at the edges of the mouth. Because SoftForm™ doesn't bind with the body, however, some dissatisfied patients opt to have it replaced with the newer, softer (and tapered) version, if this is a problem. (As Dr Fredric Brandt commented in 1997, meanwhile, 'It's a relatively new science; until we've treated hundreds of thousands of people, we won't really know about things like irritation, scars at the incision sites or whether the product will shift sometime down the road.' Again, this illustrates the newness of the science relating to so many of these 'fillers'.) Another problem, according to some doctors, is that 'the strips are linear – and lines often aren't. They go off in different directions'. Dr Debra Jaliman says: 'If it's not placed exactly right, you end up with a line and a bump.' There's also the possibility of tiny scars at the point of entry. Dr Brandt has commented, 'I'm not saying these marks will be perceptible to the whole world, but if you look closely in the mirror, you'll see them.'

Upkeep SoftForm™ is a permanent implant, so once it's there, it's supposed to be there. SoftForm™ tends to appeal to patients who've been paying a lot for collagen maintenance. However, as Wendy Lewis points out, 'It can move, get infected and extrude through the skin – in which case, it has to be removed...' (See also **The risks**.) Doctors often recommend Collagen Replacement Therapy® or Hylaform to further enhance the effects and achieve the best results – and it's worth remembering that these need regular maintenance.

How much it costs From £600 per strand.

CASE STUDY   'I had SoftForm™'

For a first-person account of SoftForm™ as a lip-enhancer, see page 83.

Fillers: the cheats

■ Wisdom from the pros is to avoid applying foundation and powder to areas like the smile lines, because it simply draws attention to them. The message here is 'less is more'; try skipping foundation in areas of lines and wrinkles, instead focussing coverage on areas of uneven pigmentation (for instance, broken veins). The one foundation I've found that actually makes lines look less obvious, though, is Lancôme Optim'âge, which actually bounces light back from fine lines, softening their appearance. (It's available at Lancôme counters everywhere.)

■ Although, as I've just said, you should avoid applying most foundations to lined areas, Prescriptives do offer an extraordinary under-make-up product that works like Polyfilla and gives truly miraculous results. Called Magic Invisible Line Smoother, it's dabbed on lines and deep wrinkles, which are filled with the silicone-based gel. (Applied to the surface of the skin, silicone is risk-free.) It also contains 'optical diffusers' which bounce back light, creating a 'soft focus' effect – and I think any woman considering a filler treatment should play with this first. Try using it before and after foundation, dabbing it into areas like crow's feet and the furrow between your eyebrows, to get the best results. (It's an eye-opening exercise to do one eye first, then look in the mirror and compare with the other side.) Avoid powdering the area, though.

■ See BOTOX® – THE CHEATS for details of JOEY New York's Line Up on page 36, which works in a similar way to Invisible Line Smoother.

■ Lancôme Touche d'Optimâge Line Blurring Concentrate is a clear gel-in-a-wand that helps fill in nooks and crannies, leaving skin looking smoother – and features light-diffusing ingredients to make lines appear less visible. I love it.

■ Another product for softening the look of fine lines and wrinkles is Trish McEvoy's Refiner (see RESOURCES): a wand of moisturising, light-diffusing ingredients that make the area look dewier, fresher – and therefore younger. (You can fake this effect by applying a dab or two of your regular moisturiser over make-up, if you insist on ignoring my advice and using it in lined zones!) What makes the Refiner handy is that it's slim enough to slip in a handbag or even a purse, to add a dab of moisture to dry, lined areas during the day.

■ Yves Saint Laurent's Touche Eclat – found in just about every famous face's make-up bag – is well-known for its ability to cover up dark circles under the eyes, but it can also be used to soften the look of deep wrinkles like the crease that runs from nose to mouth; apply (it has a brush applicator) along the line, then blend outward.

■ There's actually such a thing as a line-filling pencil, created by Victoria Vogue. (See RESOURCES). Apply the Line Filler Pencil under your foundation, or use alone. Pat gently, and it shouldn't cake, peel or flake off. It can be re-used during the day, as needed. (It is, however, crucial to get a colour that matches your skintone – or the results are going to look really weird.)

■ Face powder can look dusty on dry skin, settling into lines and emphasising them. Filling a spritzer with alcohol-free toner or rosewater and spraying it on your face to set make-up and powder delivers a dewier, younger look.

CHAPTER 5

Lips – pump up the volume

Ironic, isn't it: just when our waistlines start to expand, our lips thin. With age, the plump, fatty cushion that gives lips their volume reduces. (Fat literally heads south – thanks to gravity.) Muscle tension and tone become lax; lips begin to hang and lengthen – as well as to thin. The result is that many women hitting mid-age find their lips are visibly deflating by the year. (Along with their self-confidence.) Certainly, a plumper pout is regarded, even subconsciously, as a sign of sensuality and a symbol of youth.

Some younger people, too, are keen to improve on what nature gave them. Blame Hollywood – and the catwalk – for their role, too. Once we looked out for an actress's change of hair colour. Now we can check out her lips deflating and inflating from film to film. Ever since Barbara Hershey's collagen-filled bee-stung lips debuted over a decade ago, women have worn thin the carpets of doctors' waiting rooms in pursuit of the same (transient) effect.

However, I believe it's important to be armed with as much information as possible before opting for lip enhancement. (Remember, fillers aren't your only resort. Some of the 'cheats' on pages 88–90 can also deliver near-miraculous, albeit temporary, results.)

Women who've had lip enhancement have told me that they feel it's very important that the doctor has a real appreciation of their individual beauty. Pamela Anderson's lips may just look ridiculous on your face. (It's up to you to decide whether you think they look slightly ridiculous on hers...) Almost anyone is a candidate for lip enhancement; you don't have to wait till the ageing process kicks in. According to Dr James Romano, a San Francisco plastic surgeon, the split on his patients is 40 per cent under thirty-fives, 60 per cent older men and women seeking to reverse age-related lip-thinning.

However, it's worth talking to your dentist or an oral surgeon before you visit a cosmetic surgeon or cosmeto-dermatologist. In some cases, your 'dental architecture' can influence the way your lips 'sit' – for instance, if you have over-bite or under-bite, or your teeth are very crooked. In this case, lip enhancement alone may not correct the problem and you may just find you've wasted your money because the results just don't live up to your expectations.

As with other techniques in the first half of this book, lip enhancement should strictly only be carried out by a medical doctor with experience in this field. There are, though, some cowboys (and cowgirls) out there, some without medical qualifications, doing this work. Because of the potentially catastrophic results if the procedure went wrong – loss of feeling or other nerve damage (think: a lifetime of drooling) – I personally think you would be mad to have this done by anyone without researching their credentials fully beforehand. There have been cases of 'ulcerated nodules' after lip treatment, as well as persistent swelling.

Details on the fillers themselves, how they're injected and who they're suitable for are featured in the FILL 'EM UP chapter. But here, I've tried to give some insight into what to expect for lips, as opposed to facial line-filling, by talking to patients who've paid to have some of these fillers for lip enhancement. However, lip treatment is by no means as straightforward as line-filling. The 'downtime' – no matter what your doctor tells you – is likely to be longer, and the pain factor can be higher: the skin on our lips, an erogenous zone, is some of the most sensitive anywhere on the body. And it's worth remembering, too, that the results are likely to be more obvious to strangers than line-filling. Even with a temporary filler, if you don't like the result, you're stuck with it till the material has metabolised. (It's not unknown, meanwhile, for lip implants to be sensed by someone kissing you – particularly if you had very thin lips beforehand.)

The temporary fillers are a high-maintenance option; the fact that we move our mouths so much probably has something to do with the fast dispersal of fillers from the lip zone. The 'permanent' fillers include Artecoll® and Evolution – delivered by injection – and SoftForm™, which is threaded into the lip via four small incisions. Small stitches will be used to seal the wounds, which will probably be removed in about a week. (The cleverer surgeons manage to snip these off almost at skin-level. Be sure to ask how obvious the stitches will be after your treatment, because this can affect how much 'downtime' to plan for.) Injectables are usually better if you want actual volume in the lips themselves – the famous 'Paris pout', as it's called. Implants may be a better option if you want to improve the outline of your mouth. (Which also has the effect of making fine lines – feathering and smoker's lines – less visible, because it pushes them out from the inside.)

Whichever technique you opt for, expect to be very 'full-lipped' post-operatively. Your doctor should warn you that bruising and swelling are natural consequences of the surgical procedure you're about to undergo. You'll probably have difficulty drinking or eating without spilling – at least for some hours, if not longer. (Not an ideal treatment before a job interview or a hot date, then.) There will probably be pain, especially if you press on them. (Another friend described tooth-brushing in the couple of days after her lip-plumping as 'agony'.) What may be more unsettling still is a sensation of numbness, from the swelling putting pressure on the nerves in your lips. (If your lips weren't numb, you'd be in even more pain, so be thankful for small mercies.)

Gradually, the swelling will subside – probably more than you want it to – but the sensitivity to pressure can last for about three weeks. As with most procedures, how badly you bruise will depend – well, on how badly you bruise. Some doctors prescribe a pharmaceutical-grade arnica – sometimes in the form of a product called SinEcch (which is said to reduce the tendency to swelling and bruising by as much as 80 per cent) – and a topical arnica ointment as well. (If they don't offer you arnica, you can get this at most natural food stores; go for the 30x strength and take it every two hours for around seven days.)

It can be hard to imagine just what you'll look like with fuller lips. (A friend of mine, interviewed for this book, woke up feeling like Daffy Duck afterwards – and it was some months before her husband stopped teasing her.) Some doctors, then, offer useful computer imaging which can show the predicted results to you the patient, to help you make up your mind the level of enlargement you desire – from mild to moderate to extreme. And – the question everyone wants the answer to – what will it feel like to your significant other? According to the Facial Plastic Surgery Network, 'If you had very thin lips and shoved an implant into a tight space it is quite possible for him or her to be able to feel the implant. But the good thing is, you get used to it, very quickly.'

Take 'before' and 'just after' pictures – and then another set, when the swelling's gone down. The reason for this is that if you opt to have the treatment again, you can show the pictures to the doctor – in just the same way as a photograph is useful to show a hairdresser, to ensure you're talking the same language. (What's 'full' to you may not be to him. Or vice versa.)

There is, meanwhile, a risk of infection at the site of the incision/injection. That's because the mouth harbours millions of bacteria: it's warm, moist and frequently given food for bacteria to feed on. Be aware that if you have any kind of dental surgery before your lip enhancement – even tooth-polishing – more bacteria than usual will be released. In this case, some doctors like to prescribe antibiotics as a preventive measure. Because lips are mobile (you have to eat, even if you can manage to stay silent), they take longer to heal than parts of the body you can keep immobile.

But as with any procedure, you should ask all of the questions outlined in the BEFORE YOU DO A THING chapter at the beginning of this book. Your doctor should discuss the treatment options with you. Afterwards, use this book to weigh up which treatment you feel most comfortable with.

Then it's your lips – in their hands…

CASE STUDY   'I had SoftForm™ to enhance my lips'

– VERONIQUE, 58

'At fifty-six, I had started to noticed fine lines on the upper lip – the legacy of living in Southern California. So I went to see a surgeon, recommended by a friend, for advice. He recommended SoftForm™, a fairly new procedure – and heart-stoppingly expensive. But what appealed to me was a) that it was permanent – so no upkeep – and b) that the SoftForm™ had been used for years in vein and artery surgery, so it had a history. And unlike silicone, there's no risk of hardening or shifting, or rejection by the body. (Although there's always a first time, I was warned…)

'On the day itself, I arrived at the clinic utterly terrified; as an actress, my face is my fortune and I was so scared something might go wrong. During the procedure, my face was covered up with a scarf-like cloth, with a hole cut for my mouth. (I couldn't have watched, even if I'd wanted to – which I didn't!) I had a local anaesthetic, first with a gel on the inside of the lips, then a massive injection to numb the whole area. He began to work on the outside with a scalpel and every time I jumped, I got another injection, so that basically, I didn't feel a damned thing. Six incisions were made along the upper lip. Then the SoftForm™ thread was threaded through using an ultra-fine needle, almost as thin as a hair. It felt odd; I could feel something going on – but there was absolutely no pain. Then the incisions were closed – using tiny fly-leg stitches (which I could easily cover with lipstick), although now I believe a type of skin glue is also sometimes used.

'Immediately afterwards, my lips were a bit swollen – but in fact, I had the SoftForm™ done in my lunch hour and went straight back to work. It was exactly like going to the dentist; within an hour, I was less numb – and within two hours, the anaesthetic had worn off. It was a little tender and sore where the stitches had been, and because of the trauma to the tissues – but basically pain-free. When I got home that night and looked in the mirror, I thought: "I hope I've done the right thing!"

'The swelling was worst at the end of the second day, but by the third day, it had started to go down, I could see how my lips would look – and I liked what I saw. I am incredibly pleased with the results – so much so that I am now going to have the grooves running from the nose to the corners of the mouth filled with SoftForm™. The results weren't obvious to anyone – but I can see a real improvement. Friends simply said how well I looked. So I haven't enlightened them…'

CASE STUDY   ## 'I had Artecoll® for a filmstar pout'

– TRACEY, 31

'The honest truth is I saw pouty lips as a fashion accessory – not something you had to be rich and famous for; it was available to all. My lips were actually quite normal – but I wanted that really "pouty" look which I felt was very modern. I read a feature in a newspaper on different Valentine's gifts and it mentioned lip enhancement: "Get these luscious Valentine's lips…" – and talked about Artecoll®. But I really had to psych myself up because about a year beforehand, I'd had collagen – and it was a nightmare. I was in excruciating pain because I wasn't given a local anaesthetic and the results were pathetic. It lasted a week – and my lips were back to normal, and I swore "never again" because for me it was a total waste of money.

'I liked the sound of Artecoll® because it was permanent – but based on collagen, which I knew I could tolerate because I'd had a patch test for my previous injection. I called my surgeon Mr Jan Stanek's surgery, and was told he had a three-month waiting list. Actually I thought that was quite a good sign that he knew what he was doing and word had got around. If something's going wrong, you don't want it to go wrong on your face, so I felt it was really important to find the right person. In fact, the surgery called a week later and I got a cancellation. Sitting in the waiting room, I was a bit nervous, surrounded by people in various stages of treatment – with faces covered in numbing cream, for instance.

'I lay down and while Mr Stanek had a look at my face, I told him that I wanted lips like Elizabeth Hurley's but not as full as Patsy Kensit's! He gave me a "dental block" injection – exactly like going to the dentist's – and then injected my lips about three or four times on the top and bottom, at the sides and in the middle, moulding the Artecoll® with his fingers to ensure it was placed the way he wanted it. It was completely painless because of the anaesthetic, which took around two hours to wear off. He gave me an ice pack to hold next to the area while I recovered in the waiting room for a few minutes. Immediately afterward it felt incredibly fat and alien, as if my lips belonged to someone else; when I looked in the mirror they were hideously swollen and my husband said, "Omigod, it looks as if someone's slapped you." When he kissed me, he said my lips were really springy!

'Fifty per cent of the effect subsides within twenty-four hours, though, so when I woke up in the morning, I loved the effect – and my husband said my lips looked fabulous. Altogether I had three sessions, around three months apart, until the effect was 100 per cent. I recently had my passport done and when I looked at the before-and-after comparison, it was amazing – although I don't think anyone would look at me and think, "She's had her lips done…"

'About seven or eight months later, I'm having another top-up session next week because I'm having a photo session with a magazine. Certainly, some of my friends think I'm mad – but I can honestly say I had this done for me. (My work is writing and editing content for a global property company.) The funny thing is that I've always had people mistaking me for Cameron Diaz but now that I've had my lips done, it seems to happen all the time!'

CASE STUDY ## 'I had collagen to plump up my lips'

– DOROTHEA, 46

'I had collagen to boost the shape of my lips – and also because I have feathery lines around the top lip, which was never very full anyway and has got even thinner with time. (I'm a smoker, I'm ashamed to say.) I hit thirty-nine and thought: "Omigod, I'm forty this year; I have to do something…" And I panicked. I took up taekwondo, t'ai chi and started to look around for other, non-surgical ways of looking better than I did. First of all, I had CACI non-surgical facelifts, which have been marvellous; they've helped restore the firmness of my jawline. (For more on CACI, see page 178). The beauty therapist told me about collagen, so I went to a private hospital nearby where they do cosmetic surgery to find out more about it. Initially, I had a patch test and when that was negative, I booked in with the cosmetic surgeon for my collagen shots. He didn't use anything to numb the area first and it was unbelievably painful, horrific – I'm terrified of injections, and it really lived up to my fears; the tears were streaming out of my eyes, but because I'd never had it done before I just thought that was normal. The size of the marks was as if a dart had punctured my skin and the scabs were so bad that I had to take two weeks off work.

'Months later, when I was discussing the experience with my beauty therapist, she was completely horrified and reassured me that I'd had a particularly bad time, compared with her experience. She suggested I might like to try collagen injections from a visiting nurse who does them one day a month out of the salon where I have my CACI treatments; she promised I wouldn't be left with a single mark. I'd liked the results of the collagen, but not the treatment. I bit the bullet and decided to give it another go.

'I discussed my anxieties with the nurse who does the treatment, and this time, she used a powerful rub-on anaesthetic, all over and around the area she was due to treat; I literally couldn't feel a thing – except for a slight pressure. Altogether, she injected me six times at points along the upper lip-line, withdrawing the needle and re-inserting it; you can feel ever so slightly as if the line's being filled up – but again, no pain. What I particularly like is that before she starts, she puts a squirt of arnica cream on the back of her hand and then each time she removes the needle, she rubs the arnica into the place she's just injected. She does half the face, then stops and shows you so you can really see the difference. Altogether, the treatment takes around an hour, because she's so painstaking about what she's doing. I felt the contrast with the hospital was very marked; there, they only seemed interested in my money; this time, I felt she had a strong aesthetic sense and was really interested in making me more beautiful. As promised, I wasn't left with a single mark and could have gone out an hour later to an important meeting. There's a slight sensation of unfamiliarity – like it's not part of your body, there's something "extra" there – but you soon get used to it.

'I've always had a very flat top lip and now it seems to rest better on the bottom lip. I've found it an amazing confidence-booster – and it's even made me start wearing lipstick for the very first time in my life; in the past, I was always self-conscious about drawing attention to my lips. (I didn't even wear lipstick on my wedding day!) Now I have a make-up bag full of lipliners and lipsticks!

'I'm a normal person, a working woman with two kids, I work hard for my money and I certainly expect value for money. So the collagen and the CACI are all I feel I need; I can't imagine wanting anything else and don't feel I'm on some kind of "slippery slope"! If it was more reasonably priced, I'd definitely have it done more often; at the moment, we've got the builders in so I haven't been able to afford it for a while – and I can really see the difference. I wish it lasted longer. After three months, it's already gone from the smoker's lines – although the lip itself is still a bit plumper.'

Pump up the volume: the cheats

■ Top make-up artist Trish McEvoy has an ace trick for creating the optical illusion of a fuller pout. 'Using a lip-coloured pencil, draw just outside your natural lip line, using light, feathery strokes as you follow the line. (At the corners of your lips, however, make sure that the drawn line meets your own lip line perfectly – to avoid the "Ronald McDonald" effect.) When you're using the pencil to outline the cupid's bow – just above the middle of the top lip – draw on two soft "mountain peaks". Here, you can afford to go a little further away from the natural lip-line. The effect is to make lips look plumper...' The key is to use a pencil that exactly matches the shade of your natural lips, rather than your lipstick, though.

■ What else makes lips look more generous is to use a concealer pencil or draw the faintest line above your top lip with a white crayon (especially in the middle, above the cupid's bow). Blend with a finger or a Q-Tip to ensure that the line is just enough to catch the light, without being obviously a line. You can also use Yves Saint Laurent's miraculous Touche Eclat, a light-diffusing pump-action pen, for the same trick.

■ Trish McEvoy takes a small, stiff brush, dips it in a bone-coloured eyeshadow and lightly outlines both the top lip and underneath the bottom lip, to make the outline stand out more. You can't see the line – but it makes all the difference in the world.

■ For the illusion of fuller lips, add a dab of shimmer lipstick in the middle of your bottom lip, and smack lips together. A dab of gloss does the same thing. (It's a trick of the light.)

■ Another trick for creating a fuller-looking pout is to leave the centre of the lips free of colour. What's there will 'travel', but as the colour's not so intense, it creates the illusion of plumpness.

■ Fuller Pout Trick No. 3: dab lightweight concealer on the centre of the lips (over lipstick), then blend out towards the corners by smacking your lips together lightly.

■ Applied just above the cupid's bow, a tiny dab of shimmery highlighter – in sheen-y gold or silver – helps give a more full-lipped look.

■ For younger-looking lips, break the rules and – with a lip pencil that exactly matches your lips – draw the merest hint of a turned-up corner at the outer edges of your pout.

■ The cosmetics industry, happily for us, has recently turned its attention to creating products specifically designed to make our lips look fuller. Having organised a 'Tried & Tested' on a panel of nine magazine reader guinea pigs, these are the ones they voted tops: Ultima II Extraordinaire Volumising Lip Gloss, Diorific Plastic Shine by Christian Dior, L'Oréal Rouge Pulp and Helena Rubinstein Lip Sculptor. BeneFit Lip Plump, meanwhile, earned raves as a neutral-coloured 'base' for lipstick that also has a pout-pumping effect.

■ Look at a saxophone or a trumpet player's lips: they're always full – and curvy. Nobody's going to take up the trumpet or flute just to have a better lip outline, but the message is clear: using your lips – exercising them regularly, in other words – is what counts. Take up whistling. Or try these two exercises:

1 The Lip Pop – Extend your lower lip so that your two lips really hug each other, and then separate your lips with a loud 'pop'. Repeat twenty-five times.

2 The Lip Puff – Stuff a small wad of tissue or cotton wool into the end of a drinking straw. Try to blow the stuffing out of the straw. As you blow, puff out your cheeks and do not allow the air to escape from your lips. Then release the air with a loud rush. Repeat twenty-five times.

CHAPTER 6

The zappers

Mention the word 'laser' and for some of us, it's enough to trigger visions of beams strong enough to blow up alien spacecraft. However, lasers are no longer the stuff of Star Wars – they've entered the realm of skin care.

Yes, it's still space-age technology. But there are lasers – and there are lasers. (Laser, for your info, is short for Light Amplification by Stimulated Emission of Radiation.) Some do more short-term damage than others – in the hope of offering more significant benefits, down the line. With the more powerful laser treatments, the 'downtime' may be weeks or even months. This family of powerful facial lasers – used in 'laser resurfacing' – works by literally blasting away the top layers of skin, sending collagen production into over-drive and, when the face is healed, revealing a 'whole new complexion', once it's recovered from its 'skinned tomato' phase. They require a general anaesthetic – with all the attendant risks and recovery challenges. Initially, the skin will bleed, ooze, crust; you'll need bandaging. So this is certainly not something you're going to be able to get away with in a lunch hour. (The results, however, are akin to a facelift.)

The buzzword right now in lasers is 'non-ablative'. Non-ablative means, literally, non-wounding. These new, 'gentler' lasers definitely do come under the category of 'quick fix'. As laser expert Dr Roy Geronemus, who is Director of the Laser and Skin Surgery Centre of New York, explains: 'The controlled effect of these lasers at the deeper layers of the dermis [skin layer below the surface] stimulates new collagen formation and tightens the underlying skin, improving fine lines and toning loose skin without inducing a superficial burn or injury.' And, he continues, 'Despite some limitations, non-ablative lasers hold great potential for patients who wish to maintain a youthful appearance, especially younger patients who want to prevent or postpone more invasive surgery.' The flipside of this is that the results are less dramatic compared to the earlier resurfacing techniques.

These non-ablative lasers also work to diminish pigmentation problems – like age spots and large freckles – and to blitz red veins. What you need to be 100 per cent – no, make that 1000 per cent – sure of is that you're not signing up for the wrong kind. If someone recommends a CO_2 or Erbium laser resurfacing treatment, for instance, the 'downtime' is much, much, much more than a lunchtime. (Think: weeks, if not months. And if you hear the word 'resurfacing' mentioned, this type of laser probably isn't for you; think of the disruption involved in resurfacing a road, if you need a memory-jogger.) So if you're after a 'quick fix', the most important question, when you're shopping around for laser treatment is: 'Can I go back to work/out to lunch immediately?'

What lasers can't do is significantly fill out lines – that's what 'fillers' are for. They can't remove excess skin either; only a facelift can do that (although the surface of skin may be slightly 'tautened' by the increase in collagen production). Nevertheless, lasers are increasingly being used as part of a 'cocktail' approach to rejuvenation. (They are also, increasingly, being used for hair removal.) Where lasers differ from Intense Pulsed Light therapies, however, (see page 156) is that lasers use one specific wavelength, while pulsed light uses a whole spectrum of wavelengths.

Dr Laurie J. Polis, a Manhattan-based dermatologist who uses lasers as part of her wide-ranging approach to turning back the clock, believes there are some basic guidelines anyone considering laser treatment should follow. 'You should seek out someone who has a portfolio of lasers at their disposal – and preferably, carries out many other treatments, too.' (Dr Polis herself works with twelve different machines, each of which she uses for a particular speciality.) 'If a doctor or clinic has just one or two lasers on the premises, or lasering is all they do, then you're going to get a skewed opinion – you'll be pointed in the direction of those machines, because that's what they've got. That's business.' In every case, she believes, it's important to shop around. 'Get at least two opinions, maybe more, if you're considering a procedure like laser,' she advises.

Be sure to check out credentials, too. (Think of it as 'interviewing'; you want to know as much as you can about the person and their skills.) In fact, laser technology is now filtering down into the mainstream – and, because of the boom in 'cosmetic tweaks' and 'lunchtime fixes', there's no shortage of people wanting to jump on the bandwagon. 'I think you want to raise an eyebrow if the person selling their skills as a laser therapist is, say, a dentist or a podiatrist,' says Dr Polis. Experience is also key. As Dr Patricia Wexler once told me, 'I've heard of doctors who've literally taken their new laser out of its box and started using it on patients.' Adds Dr Polis, 'Certainly, in the field of lasers, one wonders whether they practised on a tomato at a weekend course and you're their first living patient...'

Few doctors – and this is worth remembering – probably pay quite such attention to detail as Dr Polis, who has been working in the field of lasers since 1996. 'I not only took multiple courses, but actually flew my instructor into town to assist with my first six cases.' As with all the other procedures detailed in the first half of this book, you should ask to see pictures of patients who've received the treatment you're considering – and make absolutely sure that the examples you're being shown are the work of the doctor you're interviewing. Better still, ask to talk with a patient who's had it done, which gives a real insight into what can be expected. Prices, meanwhile, vary hugely – some doctors charge double what others do, for the exact same treatment. (But it may be worth remembering that while the big-name doctors tend to charge the highest rates, this may reflect their level of experience and the wealth of 'aesthetic appreciation' that they bring to the task.) The machines themselves are incredibly expensive and in some cases have to be rented by the day for a high fee from the parent company, rather than bought outright. (Which may mean the doctor doesn't have quite as much experience as you'd like with the machine...)

Lasering, meanwhile, has its own language. 'Full face' doesn't mean that the laser will pass over your entire face; it means treating wherever facial wrinkles are seen and where they typically form on the face – including the zone around the lips, the chin, the whole eye area. (The laser always avoids the area above the eyeball; the heat and bright light could severely damage the delicate tissues and liquid of the eye.) 'Complete face', however, means just that: it completely passes over your entire face, in a grid-like fashion. (The reason for the grid is that you don't want to cross the same area twice during one treatment.) Complete face includes even skin that does not have visible wrinkles.

Some questions to ask before you make your decision about whether – and where – to have your treatment include:

- What are the qualifications of the person giving the treatment? What licence does he/she hold?
- Ask if they have been on a laser training course and ask to see the certificate. (Note the date of the course, if there is one; if the person who's going to be zapping you just finished their course a fortnight ago, this may not bode well.)
- Ask to see before-and-after pictures of their previous work.
- Ask to speak to a satisfied patient.
- Check how many treatments have been done and what percentage were considered a success.

Certain precautions also definitely apply. You should not have a non-ablative laser treatment on the affected area if you are suffering from: undiagnosed lesions, recent herpes outbreaks, warts, active, weeping acne, active rosacea, unstable diabetes or auto-immune system

..., my anxiety about
... ...ng-term effects on the deeper
... ...e know that UV light damages the skin, speeding
... ...d these intense treatments do the same? (Twenty years
... ...mber, we were being reassured that sunbeds were safer than
sun exposure. Now we know that's not true.) Or even, just possibly,
could lasers trigger skin cancer somewhere down the line? (Laser
treatment avoids moles, for just that reason.) The bottom line is:
nobody knows 100 per cent that it can't. Yet. (No matter how reassuring
a doc might be on the subject.) And it's just something that you should
weigh up in your own mind before allowing yourself to be zapped...

Yes, lasers have been in medical use for around thirty years – but
some of these cosmetic lasers are very new. Professor Jack Hawk,
spokesperson for the British Association of Dermatologists, believes
that these 'soft lasers' are unlikely to do any harm. 'They are an
"insult" to skin, not an "injury",' says Dr Andrew Weber of the
Richmond Clinic. But what will women who've had this done look
like in thirty years' time? Worse, maybe, than they might have done

applied – and can certainly be requ...

protective cooling 'cryogen' spray is applied to the

the COOLTOUCH® to pass through the upper lay...

(supposedly harmlessly), to stimulate the cells deep be...

surface into producing collagen. The cooling spray is vital; it protects

the epidermis (outer skin) from any damage caused by over-heating.

The skin is then 'zapped' with the laser, with a small area being treated

each time. Over the next few weeks and months, as one patient put it,

'You can see as your skin gradually rebuilds from the inside.'

Suitable for

COOLTOUCH® is most effective on specific areas of the face like upper lip lines and lower eyelid areas, where skin has become less elastic; it's also useful for softening the appearance of scars. Dr Tina Alster, at the Washington Institute of Dermatologic Laser Surgery, reports that 'COOLTOUCH® is ideally used as part of a total skincare maintenance programme in combination with active skin care and complements other procedures such as microdermabrasion, or for maintenance after carbon dioxide or Erbium resurfacing'. (NB These last two are definitely not lunchtime fixes.)

Not suitable for The COOLTOUCH® wavelength bypasses the melanin in the skin so it can be used on all skintypes – from the fairest (type I) to the darkest (type VI). It should be avoided by patients taking Roaccutane, or with active cold sores, eczema or psoriasis; lasers are not suitable for use on pregnant women. It can't be used on active acne – but it is effective on acne scars. The laser can't be used on tattooed skin.

Recovery time You may feel and look a little red and hot for an hour or two, but you should be able to apply make-up and go. One patient I spoke to, however, suffers small water-blister-like eruptions around her mouth after each treatment, 'which take a good ten days to subside,' she tells me.

The risks In the wrong hands, all lasers can burn the skin – they are powerful tools. However, the manufacturers assure me that COOLTOUCH® has a 'smart hand-piece', with a sensor that can determine the patient's skin temperature at every stage of treatment, and is adjusted as the treatment progresses if there's any risk of over-heating the skin.

Upkeep The recommended initial treatment programme is three to six procedures of about ten to twenty minutes each (depending on the degree of wrinkling you have); many see results after the second or third treatment. These are normally spaced about four to six weeks apart, in the beginning. Prescriptions for maintenance vary wildly – some sources say every six to twelve months, some say every eight to twelve weeks. So ask. As one dermatologist told me, 'You need to keep this up for as long as you would like to hold back the hands of time – or until you feel the need for a more aggressive treatment, such as laser resurfacing or a facelift.'

How much it costs From approximately £400 per treatment.

NB COOLTOUCH® have introduced a new-generation laser, which applies the cryogen spray immediately after treatment, rather than before, to cool the skin down – this is referred to as 'thermal quenching'. It also has a larger 'head' so that similar results can be achieved in less time – because the area of skin to be 'zapped' is bigger each time. The top dermatologists will be quick off the mark to invest in the new machine, but expect the first-generation COOLTOUCH® lasers to be in use for some while yet.

CASE STUDY   'I had COOLTOUCH®

– ARLINE, 50

'I am a working, professional woman and I had my daughter rather late, so I wanted to look like her mother – not her grandmother! I have very fair skin, and I noticed my pores were becoming enlarged, I was developing fine lines – and I wanted to see if my skin could look fresher and better, and if I could get any improvement in the colour, which had become rather dull. I just wasn't thrilled with the way I was looking. To be honest, I wasn't at all clear about what could be achieved, but my doctor – Dr Polis – suggested COOLTOUCH®.

'This was a world away from some laser treatment I'd had in the past, for the area under the eyes. That was very traumatic – horrendous. For a week I looked like I'd been in a fire, and I couldn't go out. The COOLTOUCH® treatment is infinitely gentler. I was given a stress ball to squeeze if the pain got bad, and put on goggles to protect my eyes. The skin had been numbed with Novocaine cream, but there was still definitely some sensation. In fact, the pain was fairly minor except in a couple of areas that tend to be particularly sensitive – around the lips, like tiny little pin-pricks.

'I had my whole face done, with the COOLTOUCH® machine

moving just a little way each time, covering the whole area. It's over very quickly – just five or ten minutes. I put on an ice pack for a few minutes, but when I looked in the mirror after fifteen minutes, my skin was hardly red at all. (And my fair, sensitive skin often reacts badly, so this is quite something.)

'Altogether I have had seven treatments – six in a row, one a month, and one four or five months later, as a touch-up. For the first three months, it was just faith that kept me going – because, as Dr Polis predicted, I really couldn't see any improvement. After the third treatment, though, patience paid off: the colour had improved, and fine lines and wrinkles had begun to disappear, as if the skin had begun to re-build from the inside. I can best describe the improvements in the words of friends: "You look glowing". People who haven't seen me in a while, in particular, tend to comment that I look ten years younger. I walked into a Japanese restaurant I go to recently, and the manager said, "What have you done to yourself? You look terrific." My skin looks dewy and fresh like a young skin, and I now wear much less make-up.

'COOLTOUCH® did a great job on the fine lines – which are basically invisible now; I certainly can't see them. On the deeper lines – such as the nose-to-mouth grooves – it really didn't do anything, though – but it doesn't matter, because the overall effect is so impressive. I feel young at heart, but before COOLTOUCH®, I'd definitely got to the stage where the reflection in the mirror didn't match how I felt inside. It still doesn't – I feel about thirty-two! – but I look like I'm in my early forties, tops. Certainly not fifty and counting...'

NLite™

The low-down NLite™ is considered gentle enough that for most people a spot test is usually unnecessary – but you should discuss this at your consultation to find out whether your skintype or background suggests a test might be a good idea. Via a high-density, focussed beam, the yellow light of the NLite™ laser penetrates the skin's surface (epidermis), and heats up the tissue underneath (subcutaneous tissue, or dermis), stimulating the body's fibroblasts so that they produce collagen. Because of the stimulation, the skin's collagen production is stepped up, gradually helping to improve the appearance of fine lines and wrinkles, and peaking four months after treatment. (Lab studies during the past five years have established that within seventy-two hours after the first session, collagen synthesis actually doubles.) During the procedure itself, if you have a low pain threshold, the area may be numbed first with local anaesthetic (usually a liquid anaesthetic) – although most people describe the sensation as warm, with an occasional 'pin-prick' or sting, rather than actual pain. The wand is placed over the area to be treated and light delivered along the length of the wrinkle. Sessions can last from fifteen minutes to an hour, depending on the area needing treatment. NB Some doctors recommend the use of Retin-A for at least six weeks beforehand, to thicken the dermis and to improve the formation of blood vessels, but you should discuss this with a your chosen doctor/dermatologist.

Suitable for Light-to-medium skinned women (and men) who have crow's feet, frown-lines and wrinkles created by facial movements such as smiling; the NLite™ can also be used on neck skin, and to treat folliculitis (inflamed hair follicles on the face, most usually in men, commonly linked to shaving). There is currently a trial being carried out (organised by Focus Laser, in London), looking at the role of NLite™ in tackling acne; the wavelength used by the laser also works to 'zap' the bacteria in the skin.

Not suitable for African, Mediterranean or Asian skins may need to have a spot test before treatment goes ahead to ensure that there's no risk of hyperpigmentation, hypopigmentation, keloid scarring or other lesions.

Recovery time   There can be slight swelling, although this is reported as 'rare'; gentle icing should remove any post-operative discomfort. It will usually be three months, however, before the effect of the first treatment is fully evident.

The risks   On sensitive skins that bruise easily, the laser can leave a small bruise, anywhere from the size of a pin-prick to a pencil-end eraser. These will show up immediately – and can be obvious in a grid-like pattern. Observes Dr Andrew Weber of the Richmond Clinic, 'On necks, the bruising can be quite bad – as if you've been garotted.' If turned up too high, there is a risk that the laser can cause blistering and purple discoloration, as well as bleeding, so you must feel confident in the skill of the operator.

Upkeep   In general, two to three sessions are recommended – but it varies from patient to patient; you should leave at least two weeks between appointments. It's warned that 'if your skin is very thin, there may be no improvement whatsoever'.

How much it costs   From approximately £600 for just the eyes to £1200+ for the full face and neck.

CASE STUDY   'I had NLite™ Laser treatment'

– SHEILA, 49

'I noticed that I was definitely looking more drawn, not only with lines around my eyes but vertical lines starting to appear on the face. I'd done a course of Eva Fraser's facial exercises and I did find these very helpful, but because you have to do them every day, in a busy life it's not always easy to keep the programme up. I knew someone else who had NLite™ treatment and I was very impressed by the dramatic improvement she'd experienced. She literally looked ten years younger.

'I am a peridontist – a dentist specialising in gum problems – so I am naturally cautious about how effective treatments are, and try to read up as much about them as possible; I'm sceptical about many quick fixes. We use collagen injections in gum treatments, for instance – collagen is lost from ageing gums just as it is elsewhere on the face – but I know from personal observation of patients that when it's injected, it doesn't last, because the body metabolises it quite quickly. I also worry about the fact that collagen products come from pigs and cows, because of the anxieties about infection from foreign proteins; those products are screened for BSE – but could there be other diseases that we don't know to look for yet? In any case, I liked the idea that the NLite™ stimulates the fibroblasts to increase the body's own production of collagen – and I liked the idea of no downtime. If I was to take a week off work, it would cost me a lot of money.

'Because I'd thoroughly researched the NLite™ treatment before I went along and had talked in depth to my friend, I had the consultation and laser combined in one appointment. For the treatment itself, I had to put on some goggles, while lying flat, before the therapist started to move the NLite™ wand across my face. It's a pen-shaped wand with a tip around the size of a Magic Marker. Beginning on the forehead, it moves across, touching around six or seven points on the way and giving off a beam of intense light each time. I certainly wouldn't describe the sensation as painful – I'm in the pain business, after all – but there's a feeling of a little heat. I've had electrolysis for upper lip hair and I can say that it's nothing like as painful as that; I found that so excruciating that I would actually anaesthetise myself before I had the treatment carried out. The NLite™ treatment is certainly no more uncomfortable than going to the hairdresser. It's possible to talk throughout – in my case I asked questions – except when they're working around the lips. Treatment took no more than twenty minutes, and covered the entire area right down to the shoulder blades. Afterwards, I suffered from a little redness mostly on my neck, where I had particularly bad sun damage (because I'm not so good about wearing sun protection there), but also on a couple of points on my face; there seemed to be no logic as to why those particular spots. It was easily covered with make-up, and lasted around three days, maximum.

'I noticed an improvement even before I went for the second visit ten days later. It was quite bizarre: if I screwed up my eyes, my cheek tissue looked firmer, thicker and more fleshy, and if I looked in the mirror, my cheekbones were more prominent. About eight weeks after the treatment, the results were as good as they were going to get; my face now looks "fuller" – and, as a result, younger. That's what I noticed in my friend, too, and other people have commented: "I can't quite put my finger on it, but you look younger, somehow…" That was the exact desired result: I didn't want people to notice that I'd had something done – I just wanted to look better. The bottom line is that I'm really pleased and would recommend it to anyone. I definitely feel I look younger, and feel confident that because the process isn't invasive, it hasn't harmed me in any way. I'd definitely consider a top-up, when I felt the benefits were wearing off. But I do sincerely hope that anyone considering any of these alternatives to the knife takes the same, probing attitude as I did, in my capacity as a medical professional. You've only got one face, after all.'

SoftLight™ laser peel

The low-down The SoftLight™ is a version of a laser that is used in much more intensive laser treatments – the ND-YAG Q-switched laser, used in major skin resurfacing techniques – but at a much, much gentler setting. In a SoftLight™ treatment, a black 'activating' lotion is used – laser light is attracted to colour – which directs the laser energy to the skin. Initially, the area to be treated is cleansed, then dried before the SoftLight™ Peel Activating Lotion is applied in approximately 1 cm-sized dots to the area. The lotion is wiped over the area until there's a smooth, even finish and the skin is light grey in appearance. The client then puts on goggles, before the laser scans the area, covering it three times, interacting with the black gunk to evaporate the first layer of skin; meanwhile, an 'evacuator' tube attached to the laser sucks the vaporised carbon and zapped skin away – a little like the saliva-suction tube that dentists use. You should feel a slight warmth or tingling sensation – nothing more. Cold compresses are then applied to bring the skin's temperature down. After the laser's turned off and the goggles removed, the excess activating lotion is wiped away with cleansing lotion and an aloe vera gel applied. If the face continues to be red and hot, the gel can be applied as often as you like for twenty-four hours. The treatment works by exfoliating the skin to reveal brighter layers beneath, and – because the laser penetrates to the layers beneath the surface – there should be a tautening action; as a result, large pores may be reduced. (NB Because SoftLight™ is a version of a widely used hair removal laser, it is carried out in some beauty salons as well as doctors' surgeries.)

Suitable for SoftLight™ Laser Peel is effective for all skin colours and ideal for sun-damaged skin; it works to combat uneven skintone, minimise the appearance of pores, brighten and clarify the complexion, as well as removing the dead, dull surface cells.

Recovery time SoftLight™ Laser Peel can be carried out in a lunch hour; afterwards, the skin will look like it has a mild sunburn, although that shouldn't last more than one to two hours. You'll need to avoid make-up, heat treatments and perfumed products for around twenty-four to forty-eight hours, and to use the SoftLight™ post-treatment lotion for the next seven days, which is designed to continue the exfoliation process.

The risks The biggest risk – albeit very slim – is of an inexperienced or inattentive laser operator accidentally setting the machine to a too-high setting and causing greater damage.

Upkeep To maintain benefits, repeat treatments are recommended approximately every six months.

How much it costs From approximately £100 per treatment.

CASE STUDY · 'I had SoftLight™ laser peels'

– RUBY, 51

'I read about SoftLight™ in different glossy magazines being the "latest thing" for anti-ageing so I decided it was something I should try – although at the same time I was scared stiff. You hear so much about the risk of lasers – I was worried about permanent damage, or being blinded by the laser, but nevertheless, decided to go ahead. At my initial treatment they took a full medical history and told me that the true, lasting benefits would be visible after four to five treatments. They explained the laser and said that it was a very gentle one and that I might feel tingling or see red flashes from behind my protective goggles, and that afterwards there might be some redness and/or swelling. Although I have Asian skin – I'm from Bangladesh – I was told that I was a suitable candidate for the SoftLight™ treatment.

'I lie on a patient couch for the treatment, which starts with a cleanse and tone. Initially, they spread a charcoal-coloured lotion onto the face which helps absorb the laser light evenly. The laser never actually touches the face but you can sense the energy – like someone blowing on your skin. Then there is a sensation of slight tingling, and the skin becomes hot. After each area is treated, the skin is cooled down immediately – say, after they've done one cheek – with an ice pack, before the laser moves on to the next zone. After four treatments I now actually enjoy the treatment, including the tingling feeling; there's absolutely no discomfort or pain whatsoever.

'After my initial treatment, lots of dry, scaly skin was shed – a bit like having facial dandruff. What emerged underneath felt very fresh, like new baby skin. I couldn't stick to the treatment schedule that they initially recommended, and had to leave two or three months before I could visit the salon again. But I still felt that I got excellent benefits: after the second treatment, there was less flakiness, and my skin acquired a new state of smoothness and evenness – definite texture improvements, as well as a certain "tightness" that made it look younger and firmer. My friends and colleagues noticed the difference and were very complimentary, wanting to know what I'd done!

'There are certain "do's" and "don'ts", post-treatment. Initially they applied a soothing gel to the skin and also gave me a post-laser liquid to apply after my cleanser and before my regular moisturiser for a week after use. I was told to avoid any heat treatments for twenty-four hours – and to be on the safe side, I also steer clear of hot baths and even cooking over a hot stove.

'I now go every three months or so for top-ups. My complexion is smoother and my skin tighter. I was recently at a wedding where I met some people for the first time and they thought I was in my late thirties! I'm really, really pleased. And there's no way I'd be going back and paying all this money if I didn't think it was worth it!'

Zappers: the cheats

■ If age/sun spots are a concern, you'll be pleased to hear that this really is the age of enlightenment. In the past, skin-lightening creams – designed to fade age spots – mostly featured hydroquinone or kojic acid, both of which have an actual bleaching action and can be potentially irritating, and they work by actually destroying melanin cells. The new, gentler skin-brighteners fade sun spots more slowly, delivering a more luminous complexion while they work. I'm particularly impressed by Origins Grin from Year to Year Brightening Face Firmer, a twice-a-day post-cleansing serum that controls pigmentation with scutellaria (a plant extract), vitamin C and licorice extract (which has a soothing action). It takes six to eight weeks to see results, but it's worth persevering. Licorice and scutellaria also feature in Guerlain's Issima Perfect White range, whose 'stars' are Whitening Beauty Mask and Extreme Whitening Essence. Yves Saint Laurent Blanc Absolu Brown Spot Corrector features a complex based on yeast, vitamin C and salicylic acid and has a pen applicator, so that you can precisely target age spots with it, then blend. (NB New or suspicious-looking brown spots should be examined by a dermatologist, or your family doctor, to be on the safe side.)

■ If you want to step up your collagen production – which will in turn naturally enhance facial firmness – then step up your activity levels; there is apparently a noticeable improvement in the elastic quality of skin among people who exercise regularly and vigorously; the skin has greater resilience and 'snap'. The reason is simple: as with everything, it's Use It or Lose It. Studies of age-matched pairs of athletic and sedentary people show that there is a conspicuous difference between the two. The skin of those who exercise looks more supple and smoother, with fewer wrinkles and better colour. (Even eye bags seem to diminish as people get in better condition with exercise.) It's simple. If you want better skin, get moving. (OK, so it's not a 'quick fix'. But as a long-term strategy, it's unbeatable.) My recommendation? Swift walking. (It works for me and I constantly get compliments on my mid-fortysomething skin.) I'd steer clear, meanwhile, of anything that 'jiggles' the face, including jogging, running and mini trampolining.

■ If open pores are an anxiety, try self-help: stop applying moisturiser in the affected zone, and pores should become smaller of their own accord. Meanwhle, JOEY New York offer

Pure Pores Serum Pore Tightener and Filler (see RESOURCES),
which creates a smooth, under-make-up base that enhances
make-up application, and helps avoid the 'pitted' look that open
pores sometimes give.

CHAPTER 7

Vein hopes!

Personally, broken capillaries are my No. 1 Beauty Woe. I've fine, fair, English skin – which is particularly prone to them. In fact, the veins aren't 'broken' at all – they become more obvious because the skin thins with age. Some women (that's me) are genetically predisposed towards them, especially the pale and fine-skinned, but aggravating factors include hormonal changes due to pregnancy/menopause, the Pill, HRT, injury, sunburn and alcohol.

Many women become extremely self-conscious about veins when the start to show up on the face. (Or legs.) Camouflage make-up can work wonders at disguising broken veins (which are also known as broken capillaries, dermal flares, spider veins or telangiectasia, in technical speak). But if you really feel unable to face the world without covering up your veins with make-up, that's a time-consuming option. So if you just can't bring yourself to accept them, there are several options for 'zapping' broken veins.

In the old days, sclerotherapy or micro-sclerotherapy – injecting veins with a saline solution – was just about the only alternative to camouflage make-up. Today, however, there are other, infinitely more high-tech treatments available, which I've explored here. If following up any of the treatments to find out more and decide whether they're for you, you should heed all the wisdom in the initial chapters in this book, which will improve your chances of a successful treatment. As yet, I'm still at the dithering, rather than the dialling-a-doc stage. (I worry that because I am so fair, I'll bruise or that any scabbing will be highly visible. And as a Beauty Editor, I feel the world's eyes are always on my face. I've had to hide away after facials that have gone wrong, bringing my super-sensitive skin out in welts – and I don't want that to happen again.)

As with every section of this book, then, I've included plenty of cheats – which (you can take it from me) really work.

Dornier Medilase™ Skinpulse

The low-down A fine, pencil-like wand fires a wavelength of light calculated, basically, to blow the superficial blood vessels apart so that some of them are completely destroyed; others are disrupted so that over time, the blood is reabsorbed – or expelled; according to Dr Malcolm Torz (of the London Day Surgery Centre), 'Sometimes, you get a little bit of crusting as the blood makes its way to the surface.'

Suitable for Thread veins/spider veins/broken veins (whatever you like to call them) on the face and legs. Unlike some cosmetic lasers, the action of this laser doesn't stimulate collagen production deeper in the skin, so it doesn't have any kind of anti-ageing effect. The advantage of this laser is that it can be incredibly specific: the spot of the laser can be reduced to half a millimetre, so that individual veins can be treated. As Dr Torz explains: 'You can ask for a particular vein that bugs you to be removed – and zap, it's gone, without disturbing any of the surrounding skin.'

Not suitable for The Dornier Medilas™ Skinpulse won't treat deeper varicose veins. It's also unsuitable for anyone with bleeding disorders or skin that's unusually sensitive to light – for instance, if you suffer from Polymorphic Light Eruption (prickly-heat-like eruptions, usually on the chest, when exposed to sunlight).

Recovery time There may be some scabbing, redness and even blistering which can last up to a week – or bruising, if you're prone to it. All of these are easily disguised with camouflage make-up, however. It may be up to six weeks before the final results are seen.

The risks None noted, by the practitioners I spoke to, other than temporary reddening and some blistering.

Upkeep Some larger vessels may need more than one treatment; you'll need to wait six to eight weeks to reassess the situation before a second treatment, as some that long to disappear. As with most vein treatments, this won't stop new broken veins emerging in a different place if that's what your skin is prone to.

How much it costs Approximately £300 per hour of treatment (but most people can only tolerate a half-hour treatment at one session, and may well anyhow find this is enough).

CASE STUDY

'I had Dornier Medilas™ laser treatment on my veins'

– WENDY, 38

'I have fine, English rose-type skin, but over the last few years had become extremely self-conscious about the broken veins on my face, which had gradually appeared and become really big and spidery – on one side of my face in particular, covering much of one cheek. It happened slowly – I don't think I had any ten years ago – but they'd got to the point where I was very unhappy with my reflection in the mirror. In fact, they were so bad that I couldn't face the world without concealer and foundation on top. They were making me start to feel my age and think, "oh, no, not yet – I'll grow old gracefully, but not yet awhile…"

'I didn't even know there were treatments for broken veins till I heard about the Dornier laser. During the treatment, I lay down on the couch and put on goggles; although I couldn't actually see what was happening, I could feel it. There was a warm sensation which would occasionally get too warm and I'd have to tell the doctor to stop, and we put an ice pack on the area for a minute or so before continuing. Generally it was uncomfortable rather than painful – although everyone's pain level is different, so what might be discomfort to me might be real pain to someone else. This was something I wanted done so badly, I'd have put up with a lot more than this if it meant I could get rid of my veins.

'Immediately afterwards the sensation was like sunburn – warm, with a rosy glow. My face felt quite tender. There was some slight swelling; the side with the veins was worse than my other side, and I had slight scabbing. I covered it up with make-up but I think it was still obvious to other people that my face wasn't quite right. I was advised that I could continue with my usual beauty regime, being slightly more careful than usual so as not to knock the tiny scabs off, which I was told would disappear of their own accord after a couple of days.

'Within about five days, the scabs had gone, the swelling had subsided – and the veins were completely gone, disappeared into thin air. The results were absolutely brilliant. I've now toned down my make-up and my husband says I look much better; I still wear a touch of foundation – I don't think you can get away without it, at this age – but don't bother with concealer now. I am absolutely thrilled with the results and want to shout it from the rooftops; it's absolutely brilliant – and I feel so much more confident.'

PhotoDerm®

The low-down PhotoDerm® takes advantage of a technology called 'Selective PhotoThermolysis', in which light energy is delivered to the skin in pulses, though a delicate hand-piece. The light is filtered to a very narrow wavelength to heat and destroy the blood vessels, while sparing the surrounding skin. The technique controls the depth of penetration and intensity of heating, so that there should be no risk of burning. To get the best results, avoid exposure to the sun for three months before treatment. (This ensures maximum contrast between the veins and the skin.) Of course, anyone who cares about ageing will minimise exposure to sun before and after any of the treatments in this book. For more about Intense Pulsed Light Therapy, see LET THERE BE LIGHT, page 156.

Suitable for Broken veins, acne scars, birthmarks, sun spots (a.k.a. 'age spots') – and also excess hair. According to Mr John Scurr, consultant surgeon specialising in veins at the Lister Hospital, London, 'In terms of veins, it works best where there is greatest contrast: i.e., red veins against pale skin.' You will probably have two appointments; at the first, a small test patch will be treated to establish suitability with your skintype.

Not suitable for Those with recently tanned skin or darker complexions, because the necessary contrast isn't there. Some active skin problems may also prohibit treatment, and you need to discuss your full medical history with the doctor.

Recovery time Most clinics insist that 'there is no downtime' and that you can return to work immediately. While in theory this is possible, some people react more than others to the treatment – see CASE STUDY, page 114.

The risks Goggles must be worn to ensure that the pulsed light energy does not accidentally strike the eye. According to Mr Scurr, 'Afterwards you may look as though you have a slight sunburn in treated areas; if you're unlucky, you might peel.' There may be some discoloration of the skin (red or brown patches), although this should fade with time. Most clinics maintain that there should be minimal bruising – but my 'guinea pig' found this was a dramatic understatement.

Upkeep Points out Mr Scurr, 'Spider veins are like weeds in the garden. If you're predisposed towards them, you're likely to get another crop, at some time in the future.' They might start reappearing after months, or it may take a year or two. (The thinking being: the blood's got to go somewhere, and if you're prone to broken veins, they'll be back.) The chances are that at some point you'll have to decide whether to repeat the treatment, or whether you can live with that 'healthy glow'.

How much it costs You will first have to have a test patch, which may cost from £150, with approximately £100 per session after that.

CASE STUDY   'I Had PhotoDerm® for my broken veins'

— SALLY B., 33

'I always had the most beautiful English rose, peaches-and-cream complexion. But when I started skiing and spent time at university in Scotland, I began to get broken veins on my cheeks. I found I was gradually covering up more and more of my face with foundation – and I'd long for summer when I was a bit more tanned and the veins didn't show. Occasionally, when I had a facial, the more obsessive beauty therapists would say, "Why don't you get your broken veins done?" That planted the idea in my head.

'I considered sclerotherapy, but I wasn't sure my pain threshold was high enough to deal with the needles. I actually experimented, using an electrolysis needle on the back of my hand, and it felt like a wasp slowly stinging me – so I ruled that out. (I was also worried about scabbing.) Then I heard about the PhotoDerm® machine, which worked on the basis of pulsed light. The blood is "zapped" by the laser and then the natural healing process – which might, I was told, include a little bruising – gradually disperses the blood back into the body. Initially, I had treatment using a very low level of light, because the machine had only been recently introduced at this particular clinic and they were experimenting with light levels. It felt like an elastic band "pinging" against my cheek – hardly painful at all. The trouble was, it didn't really work.

'I went back to the clinic when they had been using the machine for a while to see if there had been any improvement in the technique, because the idea still appealed to me. By now, the light dose had been considerably increased as the doctors became more experienced with the machine. You put on goggles, and the small head of the light machine is placed against the cheek. That gets "zapped" and then the "head" is moved a little way to the next section of skin that needs treatment. I found it incredibly painful – exactly as if a match had been struck against my face and been left to sizzle: a burning-hot, stinging pain that was quite hard to bear – although pretty short-lived.

'Immediately after treatment, though, the nurse said to me, "Oh, dear, I think you're going to bruise." I looked in a hand mirror and my face looked as if raspberry juice had been daubed all over my cheek. I panicked because I was supposed to be going to a dance the following night. She handed me a dollop of high-coverage concealer and I applied that, but went back to the office feeling quite alarmed. By next morning, my face had completely swelled up – I looked like I'd been punched on both sides of my face – and I could hardly see out of one eye. There was definitely no chance of going to the ball that night, and so I went straight back to the doctor. He said: "This is quite an extreme result, though it can happen; you've got quite a bony face and sensitive skin, with a lot of veins." I had about ten days of looking like I was a domestic violence victim, covered in DermaBlend (see RESOURCES) which just about managed to conceal it. I really questioned my vanity and what on earth I'd done to myself and felt quite angry I hadn't been warned this could happen; I felt I should have been shown photographs of a worst-case scenario.

'However, once the swelling had gone down and the bruising had completely disappeared – which took about three weeks – all the burst veins had gone, and for the first time I found myself happily walking around without foundation. In summer, this is a real relief. After three years, a few veins have come back, but nothing like as bad as before. The flipside, though, is that I don't think I look as healthy as I once did, unless I've been for a really bracing two-hour walk; it's taken away some of the freshness. Retrospectively, I think having rosy cheeks is incredibly pretty and that my problem probably wasn't serious enough to have had it done. If someone has purple-y veins – almost the complexion of a drinker – then I think, yes, have it done, but for anything less than that, I'd say: stick to a good concealer. If I had my time over, I wouldn't have it done again. Life's too short.'

Vein hopes: the cheats

■ Vitamin K – which takes its name from the German word koagulation – is the 'great white hope' of spider vein sufferers. Anecdotally, thousands of plastic surgeons, dermatologists and other skincare professionals use a product called NatraKlear Dermal K (see RESOURCES) for its coagulant properties, reducing capillary damage. (It apparently sells over a million jars annually.) Dermal K's double-whammy is that it also works to help heal bruises more swiftly; in trials, people who used Dermal K on one side of a bruise but not on the other found that the Dermal K-treated side healed in five to seven days, compared to eleven to thirteen days for the untreated side. DDF – Doctor's Dermalogic Formula – also make a Vitamin K Cream, which features other vein-strengthening ingredients (such as horse chestnut extract and citrus bioflavonoid), as well as anti-inflammatory ingredients.

■ Eating vitamin-K-rich foods may also help strengthen blood vessel walls from the inside. Pack your diet with foods like green, leafy vegetables, fruits, seeds and dairy products.

■ Since spider veins are my No. 1 Beauty Woe, I've experimented with everything short of zapping or sclerotherapy to combat the problem. The best results I've found, have been from using Estée Lauder Idealist, a serum-like lotion that goes on before moisturiser and which, used over a period of time, definitely seems to take the edge off the redness of the veins. (It also makes a sublimely velvety base for make-up.)

■ Beware of over-zealous facial massage. If you do have a facial massage, be sure to point out to the therapist that you have a tendency to broken veins. I once had a blissful – but strong – facial massage from one of Britain's top masseurs, only to discover that my jaw area (which she had massaged particularly vigorously) was covered in new broken veins afterwards. Never again.

■ Although if you're broken-vein-prone it's virtually impossible to prevent the arrival of more of the damned things, but you'd be wise to avoid exposing skin to extremes of heat and cold. Simply moisturising well with a barrier cream in cold weather can help.

■ Also avoid saunas and steam treatments, which can make the problem worse. If you insist on the pore-cleansing, system-flushing benefits of heat treatments, minimise the risk by limiting your stay to twenty minutes – and drink at least eight fluid ounces (a tall glass) of water every ten minutes of sauna/hammam-time. At home, try to wash your face in tepid/lukewarm water, avoiding excessively hot or cool splashes – no matter how good they feel.

■ Because I suffer from broken capillaries I consider myself a world expert on concealers and foundations that are dense enough to camouflage broken veins without making me look like I'm wearing a 'mask'. The key to covering up broken veins is to choose a concealer that's waterproof, sweat-proof and just about everything-proof. Celebrities like Sharon Stone, Madonna, Susan Sarandon, Angelica Huston, Glenn Close, Priscilla Presley, Isabella Rossellini, Meryl Streep and Catherine Deneuve – as well as me – all swear by make-up artist Laura Mercier's Secret Camouflage (see RESOURCES), which features two shades of concealer, for perfect 'custom-blending'. The application technique, says Laura,'is to dab the finger in Secret Camouflage, blend on the back of the hand to get the perfect colour and apply to the affected area, building coverage layer-by-layer until the characteristic redness is completely disguised. Then set with a light covering of powder.' (Her Pressed Setting Powder is perfect for this.) 'It's not a cure,' Laura admits. 'But it does mean the world need never know you've got broken veins...' Another great concealer, meanwhile, is DermaBlend, available in 20 shades (see RESOURCES), which offers dense enough coverage even to disguise birthmarks and port wine stains – and, like Secret Camouflage, is waterproof. I prefer to apply concealer after foundation, as I find that otherwise, blending the foundation into the skin moves some of the pigment and diminishes the camouflaging ability of the concealer.

■ Another excellent, custom-blendable concealer is Jane Iredale Circle/Delete. For more on her make-up (which is also so ideal for use after any kind of 'quick fix' featured in this book that it's sold by some cosmeto-dermatologists and cosmetic surgeons for post-treatment use), see RESOURCES.

■ When it comes to foundation itself, my absolute favourite for disguising red veins is Lancôme Teint Idôle Hydra Compact, which has an almost concealer-like consistency. It's provided with a sponge (which I usually promptly lose), but I've found the best way to camouflage broken capillaries is to apply with the tip of my second finger, and tap, then press the product into the skin, in the same way Laura Mercier recommends, building up coverage and blending lightly at the edges. I apply the same product much more lightly elsewhere on my face, where I think I need it – and am particularly keen on this product because it means I am using the exact same shade all over. (So I don't have to worry that my concealer is lighter or darker than my foundation.) However, that may not work for you if you can't find your perfect shade match in this particular product.

CHAPTER 8

Smile, please...

Pearly white teeth are the latest status symbols. And, like most status symbols, they can be had for a price. In fact, dentist-supervised whitening has been carried out for nearly a century. But in the 21st Century – the era of supermodels and stars with gleaming white smiles – the business of smile-brightening is booming.

Teeth yellow naturally as we age. And when we see yellow teeth, we subliminally register that person as older. Lifestyle factors play a part, too, in spoiling the look of a smile: drinking tea, coffee or red wine, for instance, or smoking cigarettes. In the worst cases, a dead nerve, antibiotics such as tetracycline or extremely high levels of fluoride in the water can cause teeth to change colour.

In the last few years, there has been some controversy about tooth-bleaching – which is still the most affordable and widely available 'quick fix' for teeth. For a while, dentists in the UK even risked hefty fines if they bleached teeth – despite its record of safe use on hair, skin and nails. The concerns about tooth-bleaching focussed on a possible carcinogenic link: bleaching results in the release of free oxygen radicals as the peroxide breaks down the staining material. In other circumstances, free radicals have been linked to cellular changes and may boost the action of other cancer-causing substances – but it has to be said that when it comes to tooth-bleaching, no link has ever been substantiated. The furore's now died down. British dentists – along with their counterparts in Europe, Asia and the US – are freely offering tooth-bleaching, which is one of the most-requested cosmetic dentistry procedures. At one leading practice I spoke to, where the cosmetic dentist sees between fifty and sixty patients a week, more than two-thirds are there for tooth-bleaching.

There are several similar-but-ever-so-slightly-different systems in use. As leading London dentist Dr Anthony Newbury (the man responsible for many a famous smile) points out, 'Think of the car world. The principle of getting from A to B is the same, but there are Fords – and there are Rolls Royces.' (He uses a 'power bleaching' system, turbo-charging the bleaching process with a 'superwhite argon light'. With this equipment, dentists are achieving good results even on stains that were bleach resistant – such as tetracycline – and the teeth can be lightened by as many as a dozen shades, versus the three shades or so that were possible in the past.) Some bleaching techniques are carried out exclusively in the dentist's surgery. In others, the patient will be given a made-to-measure 'dental reservoir' to wear at home for an hour or two each day to continue the process between surgery visits.

There's a bit of a beauty buzz, meanwhile, about new 'laser bleaching' techniques. In reality, though, the procedure is almost identical to the one I've just mentioned: laser bleaching is simply a variation of the above in-office bleaching method, using an argon laser instead of the ultra-bright light to activate the bleaching agent – although this doesn't, in reality, do that much to speed up the process as treatment is carried out tooth-by-tooth. Inventors of the procedure claim that this produces a better whitening result than the original in-surgery bleaching technique – but the jury's still out; more clinical studies need to be carried out to back up these claims.

Be aware, meanwhile, that according to cosmetic dentists who've achieved dramatic results with new tooth-bleaching techniques, the best colour for your teeth isn't necessarily refrigerator white, milk white or cloud white – it's a highly individual process. Certainly, more dramatic results are possible today than in the past – when the received wisdom was that the lightest you could expect your teeth to become was roughly the same as the the whites of your eyes. As Dr

Newbury points out, 'A good cosmetic dentist will have a strong aesthetic sense. It should be thought of as "smile design"; the dentist isn't just focussing on an individual tooth, but the whole picture.' (When bonding teeth or creating veneers, for instance, Dr Newbury uses as many as six or seven different colours and levels of translucency – a finickiness which results in a much more natural-looking smile. This is the 'gold standard' to aim for.)

Meanwhile, there are now several at-home tooth-whitening systems available – but I certainly can't recommend them here, because of the lack of knowledge of long-term risks. In the words of another leading cosmetic dentist, Dr Sunny Luthra: 'These can be harmful to the teeth and even cause irreversible damage to the gums.' These home kits are in the form of 'reservoirs' containing hydrogen or carbamide peroxide (another bleach) designed to be worn at night over a period of time, to achieve the same kind of result as in-surgery brightening treatments.

Although these have been found to be effective, nobody knows how prolonged (and essentially unsupervised) use of any bleaching materials will affect the gums, tongue, inside of the cheeks or the materials used in fillings; nor does anyone know the long-term, whole-body consequences of swallowing small amounts of bleach. Unlike the system prescribed by a dentist – who will ensure the system is perfectly tailored for your mouth, your gums, your bite – these may be a far-from-perfect fit, so that the bleach isn't so safely contained; the trays are also much bulkier than dentist-sourced versions. Meanwhile, an over-zealous use of at-home bleaching solutions (particularly those containing acid) may wear away at tooth enamel. The gums are the most permeable part of your body. Although hydrogen peroxide is a very harmless chemical – it actually breaks down into oxygen – some of it, inevitably, will enter the bloodstream during treatment. In addition, is there a chance that hydrogen peroxide treatment – whether in-surgery, or with an at-home kit – could ultimately weaken teeth – say, twenty years down the line when your teeth are starting to become more fragile anyway? Dentists say no. I say: well, at least think about it.

Veneers and bonding are options if your own teeth are less-than-smileworthy. But certainly, all of the procedures I've described in this chapter should be carried out by a registered and accredited dentist who specialises in cosmetic work. The same caveats apply to this as shopping for any of the other 'quick fixes' in this book, which you'll find in the BEFORE YOU DO A THING section (see pages 12 and 16), in order to make sure you have the best chance of the best treatment from the best dentist for you.

In addition, questions to ask your dentist, specifically, include:

- 'Is the result I'm hoping for realistic?'
- 'Is there an alternative treatment I should consider as well?'
- 'How long will the procedure take and how any appointments will I need?'
- 'What kind of anaesthetic is used, if any?'
- 'What is your experience in performing this procedure?' ('How long has he or she been doing this, and how many has he/she carried out in the past year?')
- 'How much does it cost – including any extras?'
- 'What percentage of patients have significant complications?'
- 'Will you repeat or correct procedures if they don't meet the agreed-upon goals? And if the procedure has to be repeated, will you charge me again?' (The dentist should let you know his/her policy on this issue.)
- 'What kind of longevity can I expect?'
- 'May I see "before and after" pictures of recent patients?' (The dentist should let you see plenty of these, and you want his/her reassurance that they carried out the work in question, and that it doesn't come from promotional or educational material.)
- 'Could I observe the exact procedure I'm considering before I decide to have it done?' (Obviously this – for you – is entirely optional, but you should be given the option, either on video or in real life.)

■ 'What should I expect after the procedure, in terms of soreness?'

In addition, you have a responsibility to share information with your dentist. Tell him or her of any allergies you have – to food, drugs, anything, in fact. Fully disclose any medication you're taking, including non-prescription drugs and vitamin/mineral supplements, or even homoeopathic medicines. And be sure, if you do go ahead, to follow – to the letter – any instructions you're given.

My last tip? Choose a cosmetic dentist or practice that offers the widest range of tooth-enhancing options. As with line-filling injections or laser treatments, the wider the range of treatments on the menu, the more likely you are to find the one that's right for you. It can be the difference between going to an à la carte restaurant and McDonald's.

Bonding

The low-down Before the bonding goes ahead, your dentist will examine your teeth to establish that they are healthy (i.e. not decaying). Some well-equipped dentists will then use 'computer imaging' to show you what the end result will be like. The dentist may build up a 'trial restoration' – with dummy veneers – so that you can get a sneak preview of the end result before the work's completed. Sometimes, the dentist will use a 'shade guide' to select a colour to match your teeth. An impression may be taken to help work out the amount of material and contouring necessary to rebuild or cover the tooth. Then, once the shape and colour's decided upon, a mildly acidic compound will be applied to the tooth to create a surface the bond will 'fix' to. 'Increasingly, dentists are only slightly "roughing up" the tooth, to be minimally invasive and do as little damage to the tooth as possible,' observes Dr Anthony Newbury. Layers of quartz composite resin are then bonded to your tooth, moulded and contoured – before being set, using an intense beam of light. The veneer/veneers are then polished to an intense lustre. The advantages of bonding are that it's relatively inexpensive, and the tooth stays more or less intact. How long does it take? Anything from fifteen minutes to an hour per tooth, and the whole thing's carried out in one visit. (NB Some dentists use a different, two-step procedure, removing the shaped resin and 'baking' it before fixing. He or she will talk through their preferred technique with you first. And some dentists like to carry out tooth-bleaching first. As Dr Anthony Newbury points out, 'If natural teeth are bleached first, the results are more translucent and brighter.')

Suitable for Anyone who's lost a tooth, has chipped or cracked teeth – or just wants to improve the look of front teeth. (In addition, it's ideal for people who are not ideal candidates for bleaching, due to tetracycline/fluorosis stains etc. – although these can now be improved if you're prepared to set aside the time for a longer-term approach, see BLEACHING, page 127.)

Not suitable for Patients with tooth decay, as this can interfere with the bonding.

Recovery time Zero; bonding is usually painless and carried out without anaesthesia – so you don't even have the usual dribbling-while-drinking-coffee-after-a-trip-to the-dentist fears.

The risks There's always the risk that the tooth will 'unbond' if you don't treat it right (or are just plain unlucky), but the bond is easily repaired if damaged. The downside is that because the resin is porous, it can sometimes stain and chip easily – especially the parts of the tooth where you actually bite down.

Upkeep Bonded teeth, like natural teeth, can chip and stain, so you want to avoid chewing on ice, fingernails, popcorn kernels, hard candy – and items like pens, pencils and paperclips. (NB In the sweets stakes, toffees and caramels are more dangerous to dental work than chocolate.) Watch your intake of stain-ers like coffee, tea, red wine, berries and tobacco, too, as bonded teeth – like your natural teeth – are prone to discoloration. With good care, the bonded teeth should last five to ten years, but the process is probably one you'll have to repeat in the future. Because bonding isn't a permanent solution, be sure you're prepared for the upkeep.

How much it costs From approximately £195 per tooth up.

CASE STUDY ## 'I had a whole new smile with bonding'

– NAOMI, 22

'Although I had a brace as a teenager, and my teeth were perfectly straight, I always felt there was something wrong with them that I couldn't quite put my finger on. Then a fellow model said, "What's wrong with your teeth is that they're too small for your mouth." I realised she was absolutely right; my teeth were out of proportion.

'I found a great cosmetic dentist by word of mouth and he asked me: "How do you want your teeth?" I told him: "Perfect." So he recommended bonding the upper teeth and bleaching the lower teeth. He showed me a shade chart, and when I looked I realised that my own teeth were, in fact, quite yellow. He also said that he would raise my gum line, which sounded horrific: having the gum cut away to expose more tooth.

'The whole procedure was virtually painless, other than some discomfort having someone fiddling around in your mouth for hours. It barely hurt – and I was watching TV on a screen in the surgery most of the time; I had a couple of injections to numb the gums while he cut them away, and then he built up teeth, layer by layer, and shaped them in my mouth. The material was constantly being scraped away but because a nurse was very diligent about sucking out all the excess material with a tube, it didn't bother me. It's a bit like having acrylic nails sculpted – but with your teeth. The only bit I didn't like was the sound of the polishing, after they'd been sculpted in my mouth. The whole procedure – for ten teeth – took around three-and-a-half hours.

'My teeth felt huge for a couple of days afterwards – like I had giant rabbit teeth – but I was surprised that there was absolutely no pain or soreness with the gums, although they were pink for a couple of days. I went out that night without a second thought – and nobody noticed the pinkness. The bleaching was actually worse; it made my teeth incredibly sensitive to hot and cold for a few days after I'd had it done. I went in with little teeth – and came out with a fantastic smile. Now people are always saying to me that I have a beautiful smile – something they never commented on before. I can recommend it 100 per cent. I really didn't know how much great teeth could change your face, and it's boosted my confidence hugely.

'But I believe the key is to find a dentist with a real appreciation of beauty. I have a friend who knocked her two front teeth out and had crowns, but they just don't suit her face. A good cosmetic dentist understands what shape and colour will be best with your skintone and face shape – and that's a real art.'

Bleaching

The low-down Initially, you'll have a full dental examination and professional polish. (Bleaching agents can't penetrate a film of hard plaque.) Most dentists will also insist on completing any restorative work first, since unfilled cavities may allow the bleach to penetrate into the tooth pulp and cause permanent nerve damage. The procedure may vary slightly, but in many cases, a square of rubber has to be punctured and fitted over the teeth that are due to be lightened. This rubber dam shields the gums, and tiny strands of dental floss are knotted around the neck of each tooth to keep the bleach away from sensitive tissues. (If bleach does leak through to the gums, the most serious side effect is a burn or irritation that should clear up in a few days.) Protection in place, the teeth are ready to be etched for five to ten seconds with a mild acid preparation. Then the bleach – a strong solution of hydrogen peroxide or carbamide peroxide, whichever the dentist feels is most appropriate for the individual treatment – is poured onto a piece of gauze and laid across the teeth. The dentist then shines a bright light on the gauze, and the heat and light activate the bleach. Some dentists use a laser in place of the bright light, but as dentist-to-the-stars Dr Sunny Luthra explains, 'It's the interaction of the laser and light with the bleach that creates the bleaching effect. The laser and the light, used alone, wouldn't have a bleaching action.' Some dentists continue the process with a prescribed at-home programme: a 'tray' or 'reservoir' is made for your individual smile, to be worn at home for an hour or so each day over a fortnight.

Suitable for The best candidates for tooth-bleaching – also known as 'power bleaching' – are stains from coffee, red wine, smoking or the general yellowing of teeth that comes hand-in-hand with ageing; it's said to be easier to lift the colour of stained teeth than improve on their natural colour. Brownish stains from fluoride (known as fluorosis) or from tetracycline (which can cause teeth to take on a grey cast) can be treated, but it's likely to be a long drawn-out process – up to six months – and results are less predictable.

Not suitable for Some dentists don't consider smokers good candidates for tooth whitening, because the smoking defeats the effect of whitening. (Not only that, but there are concerns about the combination of hydrogen peroxide with smoking, possibly exacerbating the tissue damage already caused by smoking.) Stains in the grey family (from tetracycline) can be harder, if not impossible to remove – treatment may take up to six months. Tooth whitening is off the menu for women who are pregnant or breast-feeding. People who have sensitive teeth should avoid tooth-bleaching treatments, as this can make the problem worse. Be aware, meanwhile, that if you have had your mercury fillings replaced with white fillings, these new fillings won't change colour with the bleaching treatment – and so for uniformity, you may need to have the white fillings redone to match your bright new smile.

Recovery time Unless you have a reaction to the bleach, you should exit the surgery and be ready for anything. (Except, probably, a bowl of ice cream; some people notice that their teeth are mildly sensitive to heat and cold for a day or two, although this side effect can be treated with standard headache remedies.) NB Newly bleached teeeth are at their most vulnerable to staining, so start maintenance immediately, following your dentist's recommendations.

The risks After decades of use by dentists, powerful bleaches have proved harmless to teeth. The gums, however, may be another matter; they can become irritated by the caustic chemical, and need to be carefully protected. In extremely rare cases, a patient may be allergic to the bleach and react with a temporary swelling of the lips. Teeth may be sensitive to heat and cold for a couple of days, because the nerve is irritated by the bleaching process, but this passes.

Upkeep There are some instances in which the first treatment doesn't work, but a second or third will. As the ageing process continues, meanwhile, your teeth will gradually become at least slightly yellower once again, and results will depend on whether or not you smoke, consume acid-containing foods or fizzy drinks (such as cola), or staining drinks such as coffee and red wine. In a study carried out by Ralph H. Leonard Jr., at the Department of Diagnostic Sciences and General Dentistry at the University of North Carolina

School of Dentistry, Chapel Hill (sorry for the – er, mouthful), after three years, the whitening effect remained stable in eighteen out of the thirty-two people he monitored. The whiteness of teeth can be maintained, in the case of treatments that incorporate an at-home bleach 'tray', by putting it in at home regularly. Your dentist will tell you how often, and for how long.

How much it costs Power Bleaching from around £550, Home Bleaching Kit (as prescribed by dentist) from £190.

CASE STUDY · 'I had laser tooth bleaching'

– ELENA, 26

'Quick fixes don't come much quicker than this. My friends all said, "Why are you getting your teeth done? – they're perfect!" But I was unhappy with them, and felt they could be brighter. I don't smoke or drink red wine or coffee, but they were still slightly yellow. After consultation with my cosmetic dentist, Dr Anthony Newbury, we opted for veneers on the top teeth, and bleaching up the bottom teeth to match.

'At the surgery I went to, the dentist had a TV that I could watch so I was able to distract myself with the tennis. A made-to-measure guard was placed to shield my gums, and then the gel bleach applied to the teeth. Then each tooth was "zapped" with the laser three times, beep, beep, beep. Then the laser is moved and the next tooth worked on, and so on, until all my bottom teeth had been treated – which took around twenty minutes to half an hour. It's a little uncomfortable, nothing more. Over the next couple of days, the colour lifted even more; during that time, I was told to avoid spicy foods that might stain the teeth, as well as tea and coffee.

'I continued the whitening with an at-home tray although I admit that I wasn't that diligent about it; you're supposed to do it every day but I skipped a few. I was given a clear tray that fits my teeth perfectly; the idea is that you squeeze the gel into this, flip it over and place it over the bottom teeth. It's sticky, so the gel can't fall out, although if you over-fill the tray, it can leak onto the gums and you can taste it in your mouth. Otherwise there's a slight tingling sensation while it's in there, nothing more. I wouldn't go off to a dinner party wearing it, but I can talk on the phone and almost forget it's there. It's meant to stay in for an hour a day. I couldn't really see the improvements, day-by-day, but friends commented.

'I had the laser bleaching done twice, to bring the teeth up to the same shade as my veneers – which is very, very white indeed, pure, pearl white. I'm fair, with freckles, and the dentist said that I would suit bright white teeth; he wouldn't do it for everybody because he takes into account individual colouring.

'Now I walk into shops and people stop me and say, "You have the most amazing teeth." I tell them they're fake! But I'm thrilled with the results. I could do a toothpaste commercial, now. Except, of course, it would be a complete con because it's not toothpaste that bleached my teeth at all.'

Veneers

The low-down   At the initial consultation, you should communicate the changes that you'd like to make to your teeth, and your dentist will tell you what is and isn't achievable. A thin layer of enamel is removed, an impression taken, and a porcelain veneer is tailor-made to fit the tooth. (Some dentists use a ceramic polymer in place of porcelain.) Then at a future visit, when your made-to-measure veneers have been prepared, your tooth/teeth will be etched with an acidic solution. The veneer is applied with composite resin cement. After bonding to harden the material, the dentist removes the excess and polishes. The dentist may suggest temporary veneers to protect your teeth until your own individual set of veneers is ready. At the next appointment, the dentist will test the veneers to make sure that they fit properly and are the right size and colour. You should be fully consulted, at this point, to ensure that you're satisfied; more shaping or trimming can be done before you're 'signed off'.

Not suitable for Veneers work poorly in mouths where there's a lot of active decay, or where oral hygiene is poor. They tend to come loose most often on teeth that have been root-filled for years, which is why it's important to share your full dental history with the cosmetic dentist, and to get any dental problems cleared up before opting for this expensive treatment. The advantage of veneers over old-fashioned crowns, meanwhile, is that only about 3–5 per cent of the tooth is removed during the veneering process – compared to 30–40 per cent during crowning, which leaves the tooth underneath basically a stump, and creates huge embarrassment if the crown falls off. (Some dentists, meanwhile, manage to get away without removing any tooth material at all, applying the veneers over the top – but this results in a tooth that's ½ to 1 mm thicker than before.)

Suitable for Poorly shaped, misaligned, damaged (such as chipped) or severely stained and discoloured teeth that wouldn't respond to bleaching. Wide-gappy teeth are also candidates. (Although would Lauren Hutton look as gorgeous without her gap?) The advantage of porcelain over other materials is that it's durable, with a colour, translucence and texture very similar to tooth enamel. (Known as 'the Mercedes of smiles...')

Recovery time As long as it takes for the usual dental anaesthetic to wear off.

The risks No more than with any form of dental surgery, but since the mouth is awash with germs, there's always the risk of an infection. To reduce the chance of infection, then, the veneer shouldn't go beneath the gum line. Afterwards, you need to be extra-diligent about mouth cleanliness: you should brush more than usual (as teeth will be more susceptible to staining) and floss regularly (since swollen or bleeding gums can interfere with the veneers bonding permanently).

Upkeep You may need one or two appointments for the actual fitting of the veneers, but unless you accidentally break or chip a veneer – or it comes loose – you shouldn't need further work on them. But veneers aren't indestructible – in fact, they're probably not quite as durable as your own teeth. You have to be careful to avoid biting on hard substances – so you'd better get out of the habit of chewing on fingernails, paperclips, pens and pencils. Clenching or grinding teeth is a no-no, too – although these are both habits that are surprisingly hard to break.

How much it costs From approximately £195 right up to £700+ per tooth.

CASE STUDY   'I had veneers'

– JACQUI, 32

'I'm not normally a fan of the dentist, so to volunteer for dental treatment felt very brave! But getting my teeth fixed is something I'd always wanted to do. I wasn't inhibited about smiling – but to me, my teeth had always looked disproportionately small; ever since I was a child, I'd ground them in my sleep, until they were almost straight across. And because the nerves were deadened by the constant filing away, they'd yellowed a lot, too. Still, I'd been waiting until technology offered me an affordable way of getting them fixed – that meant tooth veneers, in my case. When I had my initial consultation it allowed me to see how eight of my teeth would look when they were improved, superimposing an image of veneers onto a picture of me – which really helped, because it's so hard to imagine what you'll look like.

'After I'd decided to take the plunge, the first thing they did was take a putty "cast" of my teeth. Then it's a two-step process: the first week, you're fitted with a temporary plate that looks like your real teeth will, and fits over your existing teeth. To do that, they have to smooth your teeth down – which feels really strange; I felt like an awful lot had been taken away – "oh, my God, there's nothing left!" But when you look in the mirror, it's nothing like as dramatic as it feels. Of course, you have a local anaesthetic first, on both sides – and I must say, I felt like they took a lot more care with the injection than my regular dentist: none of that jabbing it in harshly. The temporary plate is then cemented into place so that you're not walking around with stumps while your veneers are being prepared, and you're back on the streets after about three hours, feeling a bit achey but otherwise fine.

'The plate is a strange sensation, like a set of false teeth, but reassuring to know it's temporary. I found it made what was left of my teeth very sensitive to hot and cold. When you turn up to have the veneers permanently cemented into place, it's just like looking at a model of your own mouth. They looked absolutely huge to me! My second visit took about two hours. The main discomfort, aside from more local anaesthetics, is having to keep your teeth totally dry so the cement'll stick. And of course the second someone tells you that you can't have a drink of water, that's all you can think about, so I was instantly, desperately thirsty. Before fitting the new veneers, they tug to pull off the plate. The new teeth feel very cold at first, when they're putting them on – and then they have to be scraped and smoothed a bit; the mouth feels a bit gritty while that's going on, like having fillings smoothed. Because of my tooth-grinding, I'd altered my bite, so it meant there were extra alterations to be made, in a third visit, to ensure the lip fitted over the teeth properly when any anaesthetic swelling had subsided. In between I had a very disconcerting lisp, but – just as the dentist had predicted – that went after the third visit.

'They did feel enormous at first, but it's amazing how quickly you adapt. Now they just feel like they've always been there. I've told friends I've had my teeth done, and they've said: "I knew something was different, but I couldn't work it out." That's exactly the subtle reaction you want; you don't want people saying, "Oh, I love your new teeth!" I'm glad I waited for the technology to improve so that the results were as good as they could be. But now that I can see how wonderful my teeth look, I really realise how tooth-grinding destroys your looks – and I regret it like mad! All those years when I could have had a great smile...'

Smile, please: the cheats

Before you invest your life savings in a brighter smile, there are plenty of time- and money-saving alternatives which you may well find effective at delivering a film star beam...

- In some cases, discoloration can be eradicated simply with regular dental cleanings from the hygienist at your dentist's surgery.

- Try a whitening toothpaste. (These include Colgate Platinum Whitening Toothpaste, Rembrandt Low Abrasion Whitening Toothpaste, Arm & Hammer Extra Whitening Toothpaste, Denblan, Beverly Hill Formula Enamel Plus and Natural White Total Protection Toothpaste, and Janina Whitening Toothpaste; you'll now find whitening toothpastes on the dental-care fixture at every pharmacy and drugstore.) These contain ingredients including superfine hydrated silica fibre, dicalcium phosphate and alumina that lightly abrades the tooth enamel, helping to lift stains. Peroxide – in the form of carbamide peroxide, urea peroxide or urea hydrogen peroxide – may also feature in the formulation, with or without enzymes (such as papaya and bromelian) that slow down the build-up of 'pellicle' – the protein-containing layer of saliva that forms on teeth within a minute of brushing. With daily use, this type of toothpaste can fade mild food and nicotine stains by up to two shades. (Although they won't work on dark tetracycline stains.)

■ Eat tooth-friendly foods including raw vegetables and plain yoghurt.

■ Avoid tooth-stainers like coffee, tea, soy sauce, berries and red wine. (If you can't avoid them, drink water immediately afterwards.)

■ If you must drink sodas, sip them through a straw, which reduces their potential to damage teeth.

■ Are you sitting around waiting for your whitening toothpaste to work? You can get a brighter, whiter smile in ten seconds – by choosing the right lipstick. According to Hollywood make-up artist Collier Strong, the key is to avoid orange-y red and brown colours; they'll only emphasise any yellow you have in your teeth. 'Just be sure to use a blue-based lipstick,' he says. 'The blue tones will counteract the yellow and make your teeth look whiter.'

CHAPTER 9

The peel thing

New York surgeon Dr Joel Studin says that you should 'think of the skin on your face like a callus on the bottom of your foot. If you don't get rid of this callus, it simply builds up and forms a rougher, tougher layer'.

Personally, I'd say: that's where regular – and gentle – exfoliation comes in. (And I'm just one of thousands who swear by a muslin washcloth, used to remove cleanser at night, to gently remove only the uppermost layer of skin – which is ready to come off – without disturbing lower layers. I'm convinced that those layers are there for protection.) At the same time, if you avoid the sun – staying in the shade where possible and wearing an SPF15 moisturiser – then skin won't develop that familiar 'callused' look to protect itself.

Nevertheless, stronger exfoliation treatments – carried out in salons or doctors' surgeries – are booming. They work in one of two ways: by using acids to peel away the top layers of skin – or by abrading it, a little like 'sandblasting'. The ones I've focussed on here are, like the lasers and light therapies mentioned elsewhere in the book, 'non-ablative' – i.e., non-wounding.

Acid peels work by removing the dead layer of cells which accumulate on the skin's surface, creating that familiar dry, mottled and sometimes coarse look; they can also work to remove sun spots, while very fine lines are, literally, peeled way. In the bad old days, these peels – usually 'phenol peels' – carried a real risk of permanent scarring and left the patient looking severely sunburned for weeks. (Your options: hide away. Or hide your head under a paper bag...) But this is just another area where the lines between medicine and cosmetics are being blurred, and where treatments have been improved and adapted to cater to our demands for quick-fix, I-want-to-be-back-at-my-desk-for-a-three-pm-meeting-type choices. Today, much milder peels are available. (Although inevitably there's a trade-off: a milder peel = less dramatic results than with the deeper peels.)

Now for the science bit. According to Dr Mark G. Rubin, an associate clinical professor of dermatology at the University of California at San Diego, 'A chemical peel is an accelerated form of exfoliation perfected to improve the quality and appearance of the skin. In a very superficial peel, there is thinning or removal of the stratum corneum – the topmost layer of skin. The peeling is microscopic; the patient does not actually see anything happening. In a superficial peel, there is thinning or removal of part or all of the epidermis.' There is an increasing number of peeling agents on the market, including glycolic and lactic acids and other AHAs, trichloroacetic acid, resorcinol, Jessner's solution and phenol. The AHAs include glycolic (sugar cane), lactic (sour milk), citric (citrus fruit), malic (apples) and tartaric (grapes). Fruit acids have been around for a long time. Cleopatra used them – in the form of lactic acid, from asses' milk. But they were never used in such strong concentrations until very recently.

And while the names may conjure up visions of the farm, the fruit acid used in physicians' offices and beauty salons is mostly laboratory-created. In cosmetics, AHAs are usually used in 2–10 per cent concentrations. Cosmetologists usually use concentrations of 30–50 per cent plus for salon peels. The higher the concentration of acid and the longer it's left on, the more aggressive its action and the deeper the peel. Precisely because there are so many different peels (far too many for me to report on individually in this book, although I've focussed on some of the best-known), it can be baffling to choose between them. The really important thing, while shopping around for a peel, is to ask the doctor or salon absolutely straight whether or not you'll look normal enough to go back to work that day if you have this treatment. You'd better be 100 per cent certain that the technique you're contemplating really is one of the 'lunchtime' options. What I've discovered is that much of the promotional literature promises 'quicker recovery' – but start asking questions and you'll find out that 'quicker' is relative: a week or two, compared to a month or two with the phenol peels of yesteryear. So if you go in asking for a peel, without being more specific, you might just risk getting a treatment that forces you to hide away to recover – when you were anticipating being gorgeous enough to go on a long-planned hot date that same night. The safest option is the 'very superficial peel' – but be aware that for visible longer-term improvements, you'll have to sign up for a course of these.

You may be wondering: could repeated dissolving or abrading of my skin's outer layer eventually cause it to... run out? According to experts, that's 'not possible'; skin cells generated deep in the dermis rise through the epidermis and shed every thirty days in a continuous growth cycle. (Although that growth cycle naturally slows down, as we age.) There have been some concerns, meanwhile, that by removing the upper layers of the skin, the lower layers will be more vulnerable to sun damage – perhaps turbo-charging the ageing process, in future. The simple equation is, 'fewer layers = less protection.' But as Mary MacDonald of MD Formulations – creators of one of the most widely used peel systems – explained to me, 'In a fresh, young skin, there are about fifteen layers of skin. Removing those would leave skin more vulnerable. A weatherbeaten, older skin, however, might have as many as forty layers of skin.' (Hence the leathery look.) 'Even if you removed twenty layers, the skin would be adequately protected.' The key, though – if you can't afford serious 'downtime' – is to take a softly, softly approach to removing those layers.

Like the very superficial peels, microdermabrasion removes the top layers of skin, revealing newer, fresher skin underneath – and requires minimal downtime. (It's also sometimes known as 'particle resurfacing' or 'epidermabrasion'.) Think of a sandblaster, followed by a vacuum cleaner, and you have the general idea of microdermabrasion. Again, the terminology is key, here: microdermabrasion, if you want to be back at your desk immediately afterwards. Dermabrasion is a much more invasive technique that may leave skin red, raw, inflamed – and keeps you out of circulation while it recovers.

But just to confuse matters further, some of the microdermabrasion systems actually have names like 'Power Peel', 'Smart Peel', 'Parisian Peel', 'Derma Peel', 'Microderm Peel'. You need to establish, then, whether the 'peel' that's being suggested to you refers to a type of sandblasting – or the use of chemicals. How to choose between microdermabrasion versus a chemical peel? If you go to a salon/surgeon who offers both, of course, they're more likely to prescribe the right treatment for you.

As usual, with all of the techniques in this section, my advice – as with 'fillers' – is to shop around and to ask to speak to/meet patients who've had it done, so you can establish how long recovery really is, and to gather printed info about the system used, take it home and do your homework. That's how to avoid being 'a walking mistake '...

Microdermabrasion

(The widely-used systems that I have focussed on here are called CRYSTAL CLEAR® and Bioskin-Las).

The low-down Via a highly controlled, sterile and disposable hand-piece, an extremely focused stream of fine, sand-like aluminium oxide crystals is passed across the affected (wrinkled or discoloured) area. Layer by layer, the speed and abrasive nature of the crystals delicately removes only the dead skin cells, smoothing surface lines and helping to remove age spots. The crystals are then vacuumed back up with the exfoliated layers of skin. At the same time, the procedure stimulates the production of new cells and collagen in the deeper layers of the dermis. Microdermabrasion shouldn't hurt – but it may sting a little around the eye area. How long does it take? Anything from ten minutes to an hour per treatment. (The CRYSTAL CLEAR® treatments take half an hour, and incorporate a Crystal Clear Mini Lift Mask – a fast-setting, peel-off latex mask – as a final step, to calm the skin right down, while smoothing and moisturising it.) Another spin on the CRYSTAL CLEAR® treatment is available: Crystal Clear Peel & Lift; by using the vacuum function after the exfoliation treatment, the face's muscles are given a workout rather like isometric exercise – giving an instant 'lift' to the cheekbone area, jawline and upper eyebrow; by working on the lymphatic drainage points, the lymph flow is also improved – helping to eliminate puffiness. In Bioskin-Las treatment, a very mild laser is used as part of the treatment.

Suitable for Discoloration, superficial lines and wrinkles, blocked pores, uneven texture or sun-damaged skin and (over a longer period of time) stretch marks. (Don't expect miracles with those, but there can be some improvement.) It may, in some cases, be prescribed in tandem with a chemical peel or laser treatment.

Not suitable for Microdermabrasion can't remove deep scars or wrinkles, birthmarks or tattoos. If you're suffering from any of the following medical conditions, you aren't a suitable candidate for microdermabrasion (at least in the affected areas): undiagnosed lesions, recent herpes outbreaks, active weeping acne, active rosacea, unstable diabetes, auto-immune system disorders (such as lupus etc), or pigmentation problems; with warts, skin tags, raised moles or broken veins, it may be possible for the therapist to 'skate over' the area during treatment, but each case must be assessed first. As with any procedure, then, it's vital to discuss your medical history with the therapist/doctor before any treatment goes ahead.

Recovery time You can expect to feel as if you have mild sunburn or windburn – skin may feel very dry, and may actually peel; it'll be hot and pink, but otherwise you'll be able to return to your desk. You should regularly apply a high-quality moisturiser as well as a high-protection sunblock in the days following your microdermabrasion – and my advice is to do so permanently, to protect the new skin that's revealed by the procedure; you'll be wasting your investment if you continue to expose your skin to the sun. You need to avoid exfoliating scrubs or lotions afterwards for at least three days, preferably longer.

The risks The CRYSTAL CLEAR® machine is pre-set at levels that can't do any damage to the skin – but this is not true of every system, so that's a question you need to ask, first; if machines are used at too-high power or over-zealously, there is a risk of hyperpigmentation, streaking, perforation, bleeding and infection (particularly in older skins); infection can also be a risk if the machines aren't sterile. Be confident about the hygiene levels if you're attending a salon; many components of the machine are supposed to be sterilised or replaced with a new disposable element between uses. In rare cases, faces may swell up after microdermabrasion – taking some days to subside. A tip from leading Manhattan facialist Marcia Kilgore, of the Bliss Spa, meanwhile, is 'no microdermabrasion for three weeks before going in the sun'.

Upkeep With the CRYSTAL CLEAR® system, the treatment programme will vary depending on individuals. Celebrities (among others) often use the system as a one-off 'beauty flash' before an important or special occasion (or if skin's just generally looking dingy), to deliver fresher and more translucent-looking skin, but for ageing and/or sun damage, a course of ten sessions is recommended, at least one week apart. (Two to three weeks can be quite usual.) As a 'top-up', monthly or bi-monthly treatments are advised to maintain optimum benefits. With Bioskin-Las, a minimum of six treatments is usually advised.

How much it costs From £30 for a CRYSTAL CLEAR® treatment and from £50 for a Bioskin-Las treatment.

(NB In addition to treating faces, Bioskin-Las can be used on the body, and also as a scalp treatment to stimulate hair growth and prevent future hair loss.)

CASE STUDY 'I had CRYSTAL CLEAR® microdermabrasion'

– LORRAINE, 40

'I am just about to hit forty and about a year ago I started to notice that my skin had gone very tired, dull and lifeless. In the past, I've used mud masks and exfoliants but I got to the stage where I thought I needed more help. I don't smoke, but I had a few fine lines, especially around the mouth, and pigmentation marks from being on the Pill for a long time. I don't wear a lot of make-up but I wanted to be able to get away with wearing less, for a more natural look.

'First, the skin's cleansed and toned – otherwise the machine would be using half its energy taking your make-up off! It's like having your skin vacuumed; it's rubbed with a handset that blasts it with what feels like very fine, soft grains of sand – and at the same time, sucks it all off again. You can feel the debris coming off, and if you look in the jar that's attached you can actually see the gunk. It's disgusting to discover what's been in your pores all this time. I'm usually a bit rosy afterwards, but there's no pain or discomfort.

'Straight away after the first treatment I could see an improvement. My skin looked and felt very refreshed, and next day, when I went to make myself up, it glided on; my skin was really, really soft – just like a baby's bottom! There's no other way to describe it. After the third or fourth treatment, I could see the fine lines disappearing. I have one particular line, under my chin, which I'd pointed out to the therapist, and she targeted it with the machine. Next day, the skin was falling off in flakes, but the line is definitely softer. The only other area that flakes afterwards is around the nose, sometimes, but that's temporary and seems to improve if I use the moisturiser they give me.

'I had my course of ten treatments, a week apart. You want more; you want to be nicer, sooner – but because it takes off the top layers of skin, they refused to do that. Now, for maintenance, I have it once every six weeks. If I have a really special event I'll treat myself to the deluxe version, with the mini-lift mask, which is left on for half an hour; I usually drift off to sleep then.

'I really don't look lined; I think I look wonderful – and so do my friends. Organising my birthday party, people have been saying, "You just don't look forty!" I'll certainly be carrying on. I couldn't face a facelift, I'm not brave enough for lasers – so this is the perfect solution.'

CASE STUDY   ## 'I had Bioskin-Las microdermabrasion'

– JACQUELINE, 58

'I originally went for this treatment for acne scarring, which has been a problem all my adult life; I have pitted scars known as "icicle scars" because they are tiny but very deep. As I've aged, my pores have become much larger. Around my chin, I noticed that the scars had started to form a network so that I had a very crumpled look to my skin. (I sometimes wonder if I destroyed the collagen by squeezing the zits so much when I was younger.) I looked at myself in a mirror one day – one of those mirrors where you look down at your reflection (which is always a mistake, I find) – and thought, "Hell, I have to do something about this."

'I read about the Bioskin-Las treatment in a magazine and went for a consultation. They had a very nice bedside manner at this salon, plenty of whale and dolphin music to relax you – and the treatment starts with a beautiful cleanse, as a preparation for the microdermabrasion. Using a pen-like implement, they shoot tiny crystals at your face and suck them up at the same time. It's aluminium oxide; because I do a lot of home decorating, I've checked out the DIY store and basically, it's the same stuff as in sandpaper. The sensation is a light burning – but I think pain thresholds come in, here, and I must say I have a very high tolerance to pain. For part of the treatment, the therapist focuses on a specific area – in particular they're trying to "Tippex-out" the creases on my chin. They work hard to keep the crystals out of your ears and eyes, but I discovered after my first treatment it's a good idea to take my contacts out first. After the microdermabrasion itself, they apply a cooling cream and the skin is pulled upwards and outwards with a light finger massage. The laser part of the treatment comes next – like a large flashlight, but it isn't even warm; there's no sensation at all. I sometimes have to ask, "Are you sure it's working?" and they tell me yes, the light's on.

'After that comes a peppermint mask which is left on while I lie back and listen to the whales moaning; the mint seems to do the trick of cooling the skin right down. When that's cleansed with water and pads, they apply their own sunblock – Derma Block – to protect my skin, which feels as if it should be looking quite rough and raw but is actually super-soft to the touch. I look healthy and glow-y, but more important, my skin has improved now to the point where I can get on the tube without putting on make-up first. I'd never have felt self-confident enough to do that in the past.

'I wouldn't call it an overnight fix; I've had forty-nine, so far – one a week, only missing holidays. I also use the Bioskin range of products which are supposed to "keep up the good work" at home. People who see me all the time don't comment on the improvement, but people I haven't bumped into for a while say how well I look. The scars are definitely far less obvious than they were; I can get away with far less make-up than in the past and although my skin's not perfect, I'm much, much better – and very, very pleased.'

MD Forté Glycolic chemical peel

The low-down MD Formulations offer several strengths of peels – all of which fall under the umbrella of 'lunchtime fixes', after which you should be able to go straight back to work; the 40 per cent peel is available through beauty salons, while the 70 per cent peel is carried out by doctors, nurses or beauty therapists working under the guidance of a medical doctor (so that he/she can take responsibility for the treatment). These 40 per cent and 70 per cent peels are classed as 'very superficial'; there is also a 98 per cent is a superficial peel. The therapist/doctor will discuss your individual case with you and prescribe accordingly. The skin is 'primed' before treatment with a home programme of MD Forté skincare lasting a fortnight, which incorporates an SPF15 day moisturiser to shield the skin. Once in the clinic, the skin is cleansed and prepared with MD Forté Skin Cleansing and Prepping Solution which is rubbed lightly over the area to be treated with a cotton gauze pad. A thin layer of the Glycolic Peel Gel is then applied with a cotton bud in circular movements. During full face treatments, application starts at the forehead and sides of the face. The central area is covered next, including the upper lip, lower brow-bone and cheeks, and finally, the neck is treated. After four to six minutes, maximum, the gel is thoroughly removed with a moistened cloth or sponge. Finally, MD Forté Advanced Hydrating Cream or Gel, plus an SPF15, is applied.

Suitable for This peel is most often used to treat the entire face (avoiding the immediate eye area) or, less commonly, selectively on trouble zones like crow's feet, frown-lines and upper lip creases or acne scars. The neck, décolletage and hands can also be effectively treated, and it's said to be effective at tackling oily and problem skin. In some cases, dermatologists and doctors prescribe a course of these peels to prepare the skin for laser treatment.

Not suitable for Active skin conditions on the area to be treated – such as eczema and psoriasis – can't be peeled. Likewise sunburned or broken skin. Patients on Roaccutane should finish their prescribed treatment six months before a peel, and then discuss the situation. During the run-up to the peel itself, during the at-home programme, some people experience a skin reaction to the AHAs in the products – which means the actual treatments can't go ahead. Anyone with sensitive skin, then, would probably not be a good candidate for these peels.

Recovery time You can head straight back to your desk afterwards, applying make-up immediately, if you like – which should glide on smoothly. You may find that you're a little warm or hot, and it's advised to avoid going to the gym or sitting out in the sun – anything, in fact, which might exaggerate that feeling of warmth.

The risks A small number of people will react to the ingredients in the peel with irritation and redness, even if they haven't reacted during the 'priming' programme. According to a spokeswoman for MD Formulations, 'If we do ever have problems, it's usually linked to the client not communicating with the doctor/therapist – for instance, neglecting to mention that they're taking Roaccutane, or that they were sunbathing in the previous twenty-four hours.' However, she acknowledges that 'in any treatment where there's an action, there's always the possibility of reaction'. The biggest risk, then, is of being so sensitised to an ingredient in the peel/treatment that whenever your skin encounters that ingredient in future, it provokes a chain-reaction inflammatory response.

Upkeep The number of treatments – and how close apart they need to be – will be decided by the consultant, but expect anything from six to eight; each individual case will determine the time-lag between treatments, but as a booster, treatments can be carried out once a month – or as required.

How much it costs From £40 per treatment.

CASE STUDY   'I had MD Formulations Glycolic peels'

───

– WENDY, 50

'I have always suffered with acne, all my adult life, and taken antibiotics to cure it. It seemed to leave my skin looking thick and dull and I wanted something to slough away the top layers, and my dermatologist recommended the MD Formulations peels. Obviously they can't treat active acne, but since mine was controlled with drugs, that was no problem.

'I actually enjoy the peels and find them very relaxing. They start with a cleanse, to get rid of make-up, and then paint on the peel – which is like a sticky goo – setting a timer when it's in place so they know when to remove it. (That's quite reassuring: the idea that it couldn't be on any longer than necessary, eating away at your face.) It doesn't hurt at all – there's just a slight tingling, and nothing unpleasant; the sensation's cool, rather than hot. All along, I'm asked: "How is this feeling?" – so I feel very much in control of the situation; if you're doing this, placing your face in someone's hands to have acid put on it, you'd better trust them... I was started on a low-percentage peel and as my skin has proved that it can tolerate the acid, both the strength and the amount of time it's left in place have been increased. I'm up to twenty minutes, on some visits – I've had around twenty peels, in all – but each time, beforehand, they analyse my skin to see what strength and time it should be able to tolerate this time.

'I'm so relaxed while this is going on that I could almost drift off to sleep. When time's up, they remove the peel with a damp pad and apply a slightly tacky moisturiser, which feels beautiful. My skin feels very clean and almost polished, as well as dewy. Immediately afterwards, it can look a little pink, but never red or raw. I always have my peels in the evening so I can skip make-up and go straight home to bed, but I'm sure if I did want to apply cosmetics, there'd be no problem.

'I now go every seven to eight weeks for maintenance. I'm off my acne medication, and I haven't – touch wood – had any recurrences. I'm pretty sure that's down to the peels and the way they've improved my overall skin, which looks and feels 100 per cent better; the texture is hugely improved. I think it also has an anti-ageing benefit, although I do believe that having over-active sebaceous glands has helped keep my skin young-looking, too! I had my children late but their friends always think I'm the same age as their parents – about forty. In fact, I've just had my fiftieth birthday and when I sent out the invitations, so many people called up and said, "No, you can't be!"'

Cellabrasion™

The low–down Cellabrasion™ is a new twist on microdermabrasion – using salt instead of aluminium oxide crystals, and positive pressure in place of a vacuum suction method. (It's been developed by MD Formulations, creators of one of the most widely used acid peel systems.) An astringent lotion is applied to the skin, before the machine – it looks a little like a microwave – blasts the salt at the skin via a tube. At the end of the treatment, excess salt can be removed with water; the skin is then treated with a potent antioxidant cream and protected with Cellabrasion™ SPF30 Protector, featuring zinc oxide, which shields the skin from damage. (Just-peeled or just-abraded skin is more vulnerable to sun damage because it has fewer layers of protection than before.) Not surprisingly (since they're also in the business of selling pricey skin creams), MD Formulations insist that clinical tests carried out by Dr D.H. McDaniel of the Laser Centre of Virginia show that using Cellabrasion™ treatment products at home turbo-charges the benefits of the treatment. But you shouldn't feel pressured to buy a whole new skincare regime if you don't want to.

Suitable for Uneven pigmentation, fine lines and wrinkles, reducing skin oiliness and acne breakouts. Cellabrasion™ can also be used on the face, neck and hands.

Not suitable for If you are already using an AHA-based product, discuss this with your aesthetician, as you want to avoid removing too many layers of skin.

Recovery time There may be some temporary redness but skin should return to normal within a few minutes. You should be able to make-up-and-go.

Upkeep Initially, six treatments are recommended, every one to two weeks, then every four to six weeks a series of maintenance.

How much it costs Approximately £150 per treatment.

CASE STUDY | **'I had a series of Cellabrasion™'**

– JAYNE, 45

'I was one of those women who said they'd never lie about their age but when I hit forty-five I started to panic. My skin was generally quite good – I live on a farm, so I get plenty of fresh air – but I really felt I needed something to brighten it up. I was looking decidedly dingy. In fact, I started the course of treatments in February, which is when my skin is usually suffering from the winter "blahs", because I really felt I looked grey, old and tired.

'After my make-up is removed, the therapist uses a really strong astringent as the base for the treatment – which stings quite a lot and makes my face feel very tight. Then an instrument that has a lot of salt in it is rolled over the face, to remove the top layers. It's not painful at all, although at the end it's a little uncomfortable because I end up with salt in my ears and eyes. This goes on for a few minutes before a thick, cream-like mask is applied, and another quite slimy cream over that. (I must admit that the second I get home, I wash the whole lot off, because I can't bear feeling anything sticky on my face.) The whole treatment takes around thirty to forty minutes.

'After the first one or two treatments I could see no real improvements except a slight brightening, but after six or eight, the difference was very clear: my skin looked smoother and really vibrant – 100 per cent more "alive". (I can't say I've had anyone tell me, "Wow, you look fantastic!", though, which is a slight disappointment, but then I'm doing this for me, not anyone else.) The treatment literally removes the top layer – it's a little like the way that the sea wears down rocks to a new smoothness, a kind of sandblasting. I had the treatments every week to ten days and feel it's important to keep up the frequency, otherwise the skin will have renewed itself anyway. I'm pleased with the results, but it is a bit of a luxury. And I wouldn't say this is something someone would go on having for ever; it's quite expensive, and after a while, you might as well have laser treatment – or a facelift.'

The peel thing: The cheats

■ Part of the huge success of 'cult' facialist Eve Lom's beauty regime has always been the daily exfoliation using a washcloth, which never gives skin the chance to build up and look flaky, dull and dead. Beauties everywhere swear by her Cleansing Treatment, a pomade-like product that is massaged into skin and literally melts away make-up. But the exfoliating, brightening action is down to how the cleanser is removed. The treatment incorporates a massage ritual which works on lymphatic drainage points to reduce facial puffiness and deliver an astonishing glow – following these seven steps...

1 Smooth Eve Lom Cleansing Treatment over the face and neck on top of your make-up. Then, starting behind the ears, apply deep pressure with the pads of your fingertips and circle down to the collarbone. Repeat the massage three times.

2 Place fingers in the centre of your forehead, from browbone to hairline. The key movement is to press firmly, hold for a count of five and release. Move fingers apart by half an inch. Press, hold and release again. Repeat across forehead.

3 Place three fingers under the eyes, either side of the nose (leave the little finger out), with hands almost flat. Apply pressure. Hold for a count of five and release. Continue in half-inch steps, working down to the jawline.

4 Place fingers above the upper lip. Press firmly and hold for a count of five. Release. Move fingers to the corner of the mouth, press firmly and hold for a count of five again. Repeat the sequence three times.

5 Place fingers, spread like a fan, under the cheekbones and press. Hold for a count of five and release. Continue in half-inch steps, working down to the jawline.

6 Place your thumbs under the chin and fingers on top. Press, hold for a count of five and release. Continue along the jawline, finishing under the ears.

7 Soak the muslin washcloth in hot water and hold it over the face; take a deep breath and wait seven to ten seconds. Using circular movements, remove the cleanser with the washcloth. Dunk the washcloth twice more in hot water, and repeat. Finally, rinse the cloth in cold water and hold to the face to close the pores. (Avoid this last step if you're prone to broken veins.)

- Leading Manhattan dermatologist Dr Karen Burke is also a great believer in the powers of exfoliation for brightening skin. 'You can do this with a rough washcloth,' she explains. 'You turn over a new layer of skin cells every day, and if you don't remove the dead surface cells, skin looks dull and creams can't penetrate. Rub across wrinkles, not along them, for best results.'

- Liz Earle's Cleanse & Polish is a cream-based cleanser infused with aromatherapeutic oils of eucalyptus, rosemary and chamomile, which comes packaged with two muslin washcloths. It's skin heaven.

- My tip for a gentle at-home scrub – because I'm not a fan of exfoliants, as a rule – is to take a handful of caster sugar, wet it in your hands and rub over skin for a minute. Rinse, then follow with a rich moisturiser. I do not recommend scrubs which contains particles of nut or other exfoliant beads. If you use a muslin cloth to remove your cleanser – as prescribed by Eve Lom, Dr Karen Burke and me – you shouldn't need a stronger exfoliant. If you can't get your hands on a muslin washcloth, buy a metre of muslin from a fabric department and cut it into four squares, or use a baby's muslin nappy-liner.

- The creators of the philo*sophia brand (formerly known as Philosophy)(see RESOURCES) are the same folk who are behind the BioMedic Peel, which is one of the most popular peel systems in the US. They've now poured that expertise into a product called The Greatest Love, a 'hydrating microdermabrasion scrub' which, while deeply exfoliating, leaves skin soft, smooth and hydrated. (It's based on sugar, which is exfoliating and hydrating.)

■ CRYSTAL CLEAR®, creators of one of the treatments I focus on in this chapter, also produce an at-home, skin-brightening version of their product, the Crystal Clear Mini Lift Mask, featuring an activator and powder to be mixed into a cooling, herb-rich cream just before treatment. Devotees insist that it does, indeed, deliver a 'quick-fix' temporary lift (with the emphasis on the temporary...)

■ JOEY New York make a non-acid 'rapid exfoliator' Microdermabrasion Facial Peel based on natural enzymes which are said to recreate some of the benefits of a peel at home – a two-step process that's suitable for all skins, except the acne-prone; like the other products in JOEY's range, they're specifically designed to offer as many of the benefits as possible of salon/doctor 'quick fixes' – more gently, and at home.

■ Let me just go on record here (again) as saying I'm not a big fan of AHA- (fruit acid-) based home treatments – having had my skin permanently sensitised to them. (And so have plenty of other women I know.) I'm not alone in this. The US Food & Drug Administration has pledged to look at the whole area of AHAs in the light of concerns that they may leave skin more vulnerable to skin damage in future, by removing its top protective layers. As industry insider Jane Iredale points out, 'They're very concerned that the public isn't warned enough about the consequences of peeling the skin and is now looking at requiring warning labels on all AHA products.' Too late for me and my sensitive skin. But maybe not for you.

■ Products with light-reflecting particles will also help smooth the appearance of skin. Check out Prescriptives' ultra-innovative Magic range (which I rave about elsewhere in this book – see page 77), which includes an Illuminating Liquid Potion,

containing 'holographic' elements that play with light to help
make skin appear more uniform, and an Illuminating Cream
Potion, in a go-anywhere compact, for instant translucency.
Liquid Powder is another winner: a cooling water-based powder
that diffuses the light, so minimising the appearance of wrinkles.
Prescriptives Magic aim to launch more state-of-the-art age-
minimising make-up and skincare, so watch their counter...

CHAPTER 10

Let there be light...

One of the 'bright hopes' of the rejuvenation world is light therapy. Like lasers, Intense Pulsed Light treatment (IPL) works by beaming specific frequencies of light at the skin. Unlike lasers, though, the 'wavelengths' of light used aren't nearly so aggressive (therefore not so potentially damaging) – and as a result, the 'downtime' is truly minimal. Perhaps unsurprisingly, then, light therapy-based age-reversing treatments are causing a feeding frenzy of interest among dermatologists and patients. According to Dr Alastair Carruthers, 'I believe these machines are going to have as big an impact in the next ten years as BOTOX® has in the last decade.'

What makes them so appealing – to patients and the docs – is their one-machine-fits-all ability to tackle many skin problems at once. IPL therapy can fade pigmentation marks (including age spots, freckles, birthmarks and other visible sun damage), diminish redness (including broken veins, flushing) and improve irregular skin texture (fine lines, mild acne scars and coarse skin texture). Enlarged pores are also tightened by the treatment. It is one of the few options for women who suffer from rosacea – which is notoriously difficult to treat; previously, treatment consisted of oral or topical medication which took time to show results and may have had side effects. (However, I did come across one posting on the Internet from a patient whose IPL treatment for rosacea had gone drastically wrong

– complete with graphic, oozy-skin photos. You should still be able to find it at http://groups.yahoo.com/group/rosaceasupport/files/firstdonoharm.html.) What impresses Dr Carruthers, meanwhile, 'is that with these machines, I can change the actual texture of the skin – and that's not been possible, until now, without using lasers or dermabrasion.'

Confusingly, there are (at least) four systems using almost identical technology – two of them with virtually identical names: PhotoFacial and FotoFacial. (The system was allegedly developed by a father-and-son team who went their separate ways – hence FotoFacial® and PhotoFacial®.) IPL™ Photorejuvenation (from ESC Sharplan) works in an identical way, but is marketed by a different company. (PhotoDerm® is a slightly earlier version of the same technology, still in widespread use; I've included it in the VEIN HOPES chapter, as vein-busting is one of its main applications – along with hair removal.) Newest arrival on the scene is Pro-Facial™.

In all, the technique's been in use for around five years – not long, in the grand scheme of things. The slight niggle I have about it? Part of what happens during IPL is that old collagen is destroyed, and the production of new collagen is stimulated. Long-term, what impact will this speeding-up of a natural bodily process actually have? The bottom line (here we go again): nobody knows.

The doctors I have spoken to believe that it is far less likely to trigger, say, skin cancer even than sun exposure – because it avoids the wavelengths of light that cause DNA damage. But by turbo-charging collagen production with these treatments, could this make the skin lazy about doing this on its own, at some point in the future? Again, Dr Hella Goren – who works with the Photorejuvenation brand system – says not, 'because it's not like we're exhausting a finite supply of collagen with this treatment. The body should go on producing collagen in the way it always has. This just gives it a bit of a boost.' But we all need to ask ourselves – and our doctors – these questions. I've said it before: shopping for a new face is not like shopping for a lipstick. Professor Nick Lowe, meanwhile, has been quoted as commenting that there is already evidence that the machines can cause skin damage. 'My concern is that these give out light waves which have been shown in animal experiments to accelerate ageing. There is also a real risk of causing staining in people with olive and dark skins. Further studies are needed before we can be sure they are absolutely safe in the long term.' (Remember: in the 1970s, sunbathing – and sunbeds – were also deemed to be 'risk-free'…)

If you're planning to have Intense Pulsed Light therapy, you should follow all the guidelines at the start of this book to optimise your chances of successful treatment. Inevitably, in time, these techniques will filter down to a wider audience through a network of salons. However, I would strongly recommend that if you're considering an IPL-type treatment, you have it done by a doctor or (at the very least) a trained nurse, and make a point of asking all the questions outlined in the BEFORE YOU DO A THING chapter. This is your face, remember. Nuala Briggs, who offers FotoFacial® in London's Harley Street, spends forty-five minutes establishing a patient's medical history before embarking on the initial treatment. Is your doctor/nurse/salon going to devote that much time to finding out about you?

Before you go for treatment, your doctor (or in some cases, salon) should give you a patient information sheet detailing the 'do's' and 'don'ts' to follow before and after your appointment. If not, ask for one. Meanwhile, here's a typical list; reading it may help you make up your mind whether one of these 'photorejuvenation' techniques is right for you.

Before treatment
- Patients with suntans (whether natural or artificial, i.e. fake tans) cannot be treated until the skin returns to its normal colour, as tanned skin is at high risk of burning.
- Moisturisers should not be applied to the skin prior to treatment.
- Make-up must be removed before treatment can commence.

After treatment

- The treatment area is cooled down for a few minutes. You may experience a reddening of the area for a few hours after treatment. Very occasionally there may be some bruising and hyperpigmentation (or tanning) of the skin, especially if there has been some sun exposure prior to treatment. This usually fades in time – however, in some cases, it may be permanent.

- Avoid sun exposure for a few weeks and use a strong sun block. You are advised to continue to keep your face out of the sun, as it can reduce the effect of the treatment and obviously cause further damage to your skin.

- Keep your skin well-moisturised. Using moisturiser with vitamins C and E is recommended.

- Good hydration is also important to maintain your good skin texture. It is therefore recommended that you drink two litres of water a day.

- Smoking causes wrinkles. It will also reduce the effect of the treatment.

FotoFacial®/PhotoFacial®/Photorejuvenation

The low-down   IPL uses a combination of visible light wavelengths which are delivered to the skin in a series of gentle pulses, via a rectangular quartz crystal 'head' that glides over skin which has been pre-chilled with a cooling jelly. The doctor or nurse carrying out the treatment moves the quartz very slightly each time; after a 'flash' of light, the machine re-charges and is then very slightly moved until the whole of the area – an entire face or neck, usually – has been treated. There are different settings for different skintones, and a small sample area will be treated first to see how the individual's skin reacts: if there's no redness, the light level may be increased; if there's too much, it may be adjusted downwards. The light itself is attracted by coloured pigment in red veins, or brown discoloration. When the pulsed light is absorbed by the redness of the vein or the melanin of brown pigmentation, it is converted into heat, and when the required temperature is reached it destroys the target, without damaging the surrounding tissue. The blood (in the case of spider veins) or the melanin (in the case of sun spots etc) is gradually reabsorbed by the body's natural healing mechanism; initially, the skin may get redder and/or darker, but this is said to be a sign 'that the process is working', and the discoloration usually fades quickly – sometimes within hours. (See also **Risks**, below.) Recent studies show that fine lines, enlarged pores and roughness are also improved by the process, which stimulates collagen production deeper in the dermis. IPL is usually carried out without any anaesthetic, although if you have a particularly low pain threshold, you can ask for one.

Suitable for

Intense Pulsed Light therapy can be used (see above) for reducing pigmentation (age/sun spots, large freckles), to stimulate collagen production and to treat red veins. It can also reduce the redness associated with rosacea, or following laser resurfacing. It is one of the few treatments that's appropriate for the very fine skin on the chest and neck – where signs of ageing often show up first, due to this skin's ultra-vulnerability to UV light. (And the fact that most women stop applying sun protection at chin level, when we should be massaging it into our necks and chests, as well.) Nuala Briggs says that 'it's the only treatment I've found for what I call "menopausal neck" – that flushed, crêpe-y look'. According to Nuala Briggs, FotoFacial® is also 'very popular among businessmen who feel that having a red face may impede them'.

Not suitable for

Photorejuvenation treatments aren't considered appropriate for women who are pregnant (or intending to get pregnant), anyone on long-term steroids or medication that increases photosensitivity (i.e. St. John's Wort and some antidepressants), alcoholics, people with light-sensitive conditions and insulin-dependent diabetics (who may have a tendency to haemorrhage). As with any turn-back-the-clock treatment, you should be asked for a full medical history before the clinic agrees to treat you – and it is up to you to be 100 per cent honest. In addition, IPL treatment may not be suitable for black skins, skins which have a tendency to 'keloid' (raised) scarring, some Asian skins or even for some dark Mediterranean skins; the doctor will assess your individual case.

Recovery time There is likely to be some redness, which varies from patient to patient. (In researching this book, I had one tiny area of my arm 'zapped' on a very low setting, to find out what it felt like. Pale-skinned, I suffered quite an intense burn-like redness with pain – and within two hours, around forty or fifty red dots had appeared on that tiny patch of my arm, which took around ten to fourteen days to clear thoroughly. If you have fragile skin, like me, you might want to ask for a 'trial' area first, just to make sure you are going to be able to get back to normal immediately afterwards – without the need for a paper bag over your head!)

The risks In the wrong hands, too-intense a light could burn the skin. (NB In the case posted on the Internet, the rosacea patient was seriously burned – on her fourth of a series of five treatments. Her chin blistered and she was prescribed a cream to prevent skin infections in patients with serious burns, had to keep her chin bandaged – and now has to massage her chin nightly in order to avoid lumpy scarring.) In some cases, hypopigmentation ('bleaching' of areas of the skin), and hyperpigmentation (brown blotches) can occur, and while these disappear, in most cases, there have been a few reports of the problem becoming permanent. NB Goggles must be worn to shield the eyes

Upkeep Initially, a series of five treatments at three-weekly intervals is usually recommended – improvements are usually progressive (although some patients will see improvements after a single treatment). Treatments last from fifteen minutes to forty-five minutes.

How much it costs From £300 per treatment.

CASE STUDY   'I had FotoFacial®'

– JENNIFER, 42

'I'm a twin and both she and I have identical colouring: very pale skin with freckles and very high colour. I do all the right things; I eat properly, don't go in the sun, take care of my skin. But although our skins look quite young for our age, I feel very self-conscious about this redness – which extends down the chest area, but is much worse on my cheeks and nose – and always wear make-up to cover it up. In summer, that's a real bore and I've always wanted skin that enabled me to get away with a touch of tinted moisturiser. I never did wear make-up to make myself look prettier – just for camouflage.

'In the past, I'd had a laser treatment for the redness but after investing in about nine or ten treatments there was absolutely no improvement at all; the whole procedure was a total waste of money. I also had a lot of swelling, especially around the eyes, which took some days to subside. Still, I read about FotoFacial® and decided I had nothing to lose but my rosiness. The surgery where I had my treatment, in London's Harley Street, is extremely comfortable and relaxing. I lay down and relaxed throughout the treatment, which takes less than an hour. First of all, she established my pain threshold – I could tolerate a sensation like a sharp, snapping feeling, which was uncomfortable but not truly painful, like a bad but fleeting pin-prick. (I was offered a local anaesthetic, if I'd wanted one.) I told her I wanted the machine turned up as high as I could tolerate – there are different settings – so that I could get maximum benefits out of the treatment. Then the machine – it's a bit like the head of a vacuum cleaner, with a crystal set into it – was moved over my face, zapping as it went. As each area is treated, it feels like it's burning, but I was handed an ice pack to place on the just-treated area to bring the temperature right down again quickly. Then the machine was passed over my entire face a second time – this time, with no discomfort whatsoever.

'I suffered no swelling or after-effects and for me, recovery was immediate; I could put on make-up straight away to cover any short-term lingering lobsterish-ness. It took around two weeks for the initial improvements to become obvious, and then I was very impressed. I'd gone in with zero expectations and so anything was going to be a bonus, so I was delighted to discover that my face is about 80 per cent better – that is, it's only about 20 per cent as red as it used to be; the ruddiness is basically gone. My main complaint is that it's so expensive; if it was cheaper, I'd sign up for a second course of treatments and I feel that would get rid of the problem completely. I'm pretty hooked now; for the first time in my life I wake up in the morning and don't mind my reflection in the mirror. The difference is most striking when I see my sister. She hasn't had her redness treated with FotoFacial®, and the difference is very obvious. She's now madly saving to have it done.'

CASE STUDY   ## 'I had Photorejuvenation'

– CANDICE, 50

'Coming up to my fiftieth birthday, I had a few fine lines and some hyperpigmentation – "age spots" – on my face, and I definitely wanted to look better before I hit the big Five-O. I didn't feel fifty – till I looked in the mirror. I knew any kind of surgical treatment that requires general anaesthetic isn't for me, as I'm asthmatic and don't want to run the risk of problems – but non-surgical options definitely interest me. I'd already had some BOTOX® to ease the wrinkling around my eyes, and when I read about Photorejuvenation, I liked the idea of how it could improve the texture of my skin.

'At the same clinic I'd had my BOTOX® done, they assessed my skin with a magnifying glass and made some adjustments to the Photorejuvenation machine via its computer screen. Attached to it is a broom-head-like device – about eight to ten inches long – with a tiny glass prism in it that's just a couple of inches long by a half-inch wide. Before treatment, I put on goggles and lay down on the couch – but I could have had the treatment sitting up, if I'd preferred.

'The treatment isn't without some discomfort. After putting on goggles – to protect the eyes – a very cold gel is massaged onto the face, to keep the skin's temperature down during the treatment, which works on heat. When the light is fired through the prism, it's like being "pinged" with an elastic band – you think, "God, that hurts", but then that pain goes and there's another ping. And so on; it's more painful around the top of the lip and around the eye, but across the cheek I could hardly feel it. I was told if the pain was unbearable, I could opt for a local anaesthetic, but it really wasn't necessary. (If you've had a baby, overall the pain rating for this is only about two out of ten!) After treatment of each area of the face is completed, the gel was wiped away; I was then handed a cooling sponge straight from the fridge to bring the temperature of the area down again while they worked on the next zone. Altogether, treatment lasted around half an hour.

'Afterwards, I looked like I'd been in the sun and got slightly sunburned – but nothing serious; I could certainly go straight from the surgery back to my work as a receptionist without embarrassment. By the time I woke up the next morning, my skin was only a little bit hot and slightly swollen. There were no immediate benefits, and in fact, over the next few days, the brown pigmentation looked much worse – almost as if the treatment had brought it to the surface. With natural skin shedding, though, that disappeared – and the marks were gone. My skin is definitely firmer and tighter, and the pores look smaller and

I'm absolutely delighted with the results. The texture is more uniform all over, the surface looks finer and smoother – and it's made me much more confident; I wear less make-up now.

'I had a standard course of three treatments – although some people need five – spaced about four weeks apart. Now, I'll probably have an annual "maintenance" treatment to keep my skin firm. Friends have commented to me – not knowing what I've had done – "What make up are you wearing?" Or "Your skin looks so lovely…" And I've had no hesitation telling them why…'

Pro-Facial™

The low-down   The Pro-Facial™ looks a bit like a sexy vacuum cleaner: a column-like machine in anodised purple, with a gun like you'd find on a petrol pump at the end. Like the other machines in this chapter, it works on pulsed light – but uses a form of fluorescent light, which is slightly cooler. A test patch should still be carried out to establish tolerance: one pulse will be applied to a selected patch, and the skin examined after fifteen minutes to check that there's no excessive redness, blisters or burning. If there is blistering, the therapist will try another patch – and if it continues to react after that, you can try again at a future session, waiting a week or two. A cool gel is placed on the skin, to lower the temperature, before the gun is aimed at each rectangle of skin – roughly 2 cm by 1 cm – and 'fired'. As the 'gun' zaps the skin, it heats up – and if there's discomfort, it can be cooled with an ice pack. After each section is treated, the gun is moved, until all the 'target' areas have been covered. You must commit to staying out of the sun for four weeks before a Pro-Facial™ treatment, otherwise the machine can 'knock out' too much of your melanin, potentially leaving skin more vulnerable to sun damage. (The melanin comes to the surface when you have a tan – in fact, that's what you see – in order to protect the skin from damage.)

Suitable for Smoothing fine lines and wrinkles, treating hyperpigmentation ('sun spots' etc), treating superficial veins (broken/thread/spider veins), removal (eventually) of keloid scars. Because the Pro-Facial™ stimulates collagen production, it can also shrink pore size as the skin is 'tautened'. Using interchangeable light filters, melanin (associated with pigmentation), haemoglobin (from broken veins) and collagen (necessary for skin elasticity) can be targeted, and the machine is versatile enough to be used on Asian skins. The Pro-Facial™ machine is an adaptation of the Swedish Plasmalite™ system of pulsed hair removal; by using a different 'crystal', this Pro-Facial™ machine can be adapted to treat excess hair, too.

Not suitable for Pregnant women, diabetics whose condition is unstabilised, patients on drugs which cause photosensitivity; if you are taking Roaccutane or being treated with Retin-A, you will need to finish that treatment and then wait a month before consulting about your suitability at the Pro-Facial™ clinic.

Recovery time There may be some redness or heat, which should subside by the next day, at the latest. Meanwhile, you'll need to stay out of the sun.

The risks This machine is pre-set so that theoretically, skin damage should not occur. However, because of the risks of pigmentation problems on darker skins, the therapist must be absolutely certain that the setting is not too high while treating these complexion types.

Upkeep Ideally, you should have five treatments around three to six weeks apart, depending on how your skin responds; as a top-up, treatments are advised around every six months.

How much it costs Around £1,500 for a course of five treatments.

'I had Pro-Facial™'

— VICKY, 37

'I lived in South Africa for most of my life and have had a lot of sun exposure; the legacy of that is some broken veins, although I don't have too many lines and wrinkles. I also have some mild scarring – linked, I think, to electrolysis. I have had laser hair removal, and the clinic recommended Pro-Facial™, mostly for the broken veins, and to erase some of the fine lines that are emerging.

'I lie down for the treatment, wearing goggles, and a gel is smoothed over the skin which cools it right down. Then comes the zapping. I have to say that compared to the laser hair removal and electrolysis, this is fairly unpleasant; I tolerate pain well but there's quite a lot of discomfort as the machine delivers a sharp shock to the skin, like a big pin-prick, starting at the forehead and moving systematically over the whole face. To cool the skin down further, the skin is iced afterwards. The first time I had hardly any reaction, but it seems to have got worse with each treatment. The second time, I was much redder, and I also had a swollen lip and puffy eyes, but we weren't able to link that 100 per cent with the treatment. My skin is a whole lot more tender afterwards, and feels sensitive. Having said that, when my face settles down after each treatment, the skintone is much improved – and so are the veins. I've also lost a lot of sun-related freckles, which come to the surface after the treatment, becoming much browner and more obvious – eventually, like chocolate-coloured moles – before they disappear. So much so, in fact, that when my third treatment was scheduled just before I was due to go to a big dinner, I postponed it a week because I was worried my skin wouldn't be up to scratch.

'Now, though, I'm pleased – if not over the moon – with the results; my fine lines and wrinkles, if any, seem to have been "plumped up" from within, just as they promised, and the red veins have almost disappeared. So I'd call it a success, overall.'

enlighten

The low-down   A pre-programmed, precise (and narrow) wavelength of light is emitted by a lightbulb-like 'wand' which is moved over the skin; unlike the other light therapies detailed in this section, there is no heating of the skin, or inflammation. The equipment does not emit any kind of UV light (either UVA or UVB), or infra-red, so there is no risk of the kind of damage linked with sun exposure; in tests, there's been no history of inflammation, redness or water retention in the skin. Like the other light therapies, studies suggest that enlighten works to improve skin texture by stimulating the production of collagen and other connective skin molecules. Unlike Foto/PhotoFacial® and Photorejuvenation, enlighten can be carried out by beauty therapists – and indeed, the equipment is considered safe enough for home use. (When I was looking for a volunteer for this section, the public relations agency handling the enlighten account offered to let the would-be patient take the equipment home and treat herself, after she'd been shown what to do. In the end, I chose someone who'd paid to have her treatments in a salon as I felt this was the way most women would experience the treatment; the equipment isn't, in reality, available for at-home light therapy.)

Suitable for   enlighten is currently used for improving the appearance of lines around the eyes, but as yet, not for anywhere else on the face.

Not suitable for   enlighten shouldn't be used by pregnant women, as its safety during pregnancy has not been confirmed. (Pregnancy causes changes to skin sensitivity.) It's also unsuitable for children and adolescents (unless specifically advised by a doctor), and for people with porphyria or any history of light-induced skin rashes. (So if you're someone who suffers from prickly heat on holiday, you should tell the therapist, who may decide this treatment isn't for you.)

Recovery time There is no redness, rash or swelling so you should be able to go straight back to work or on to a social engagement; in fact, you don't even need to remove your make-up to have it done.

The risks Although the brightness of the light may cause discomfort if your eyes aren't covered (goggles should be worn), it can't damage them like a laser can; according to enlighten, 'the light output has been measured to be well within the safety limit for 1000 minutes of exposure'.

Upkeep The every-other-day appointment schedule required for this treatment makes it fairly lifestyle-unfriendly: initially, you're likely to need a series of ten sessions, each lasting twenty minutes per eye, spread out over twenty-one days. (Although visible improvements have been documented as soon as the third treatment.) After the first series of treatments, a follow-up 'top-up' is recommended every three months to maintain benefits.

How much it costs Around £500 for a course of ten treatments.

CASE STUDY   'I had enlighten'
_____

– SARA, 54

'I live a very outdoorsy life – golf, riding, gardening – and by the time doctors woke up to the damage done by UV exposure, it was too late for my skin. I have pale, fair skin that is, as a result, very weathered and heavily wrinkled.

'I visit a very comfortable beauty salon – albeit fairly irregularly – for facials, and a visiting representative from enlighten told me about the treatment. I liked the idea of anything that could take the place of surgery and that there seemed to have been plenty of medical research done into the technique. (The enlighten person was a trained nurse, which I also found quite reassuring.)

'It's very convenient to have done because you don't have to take your make-up off; just lie down, relax and let it happen. And it is quite relaxing and soothing, in fact. A gadget a bit like a microphone is placed near the skin and it gives off a pleasant heat along with the beam of light – absolutely nothing uncomfortable at all, although I have to say that the machine itself, which the 'wand' is attached to, is a bit noisy. The gadget is passed over the skin all around the eye, especially the lined area between the cheekbone and the lower eyelid, although avoiding the actual surface of the eyeball. It never actually touches the skin at any point, but you can feel the beam of warmth. The light emitted isn't actually that intense – I could open my eye without it feeling uncomfortable, but it's definitely more relaxing to keep my eyes closed and drift off. There are three therapists at the salon I go to who carry out the treatment, though, and I have to say that one of them seems better at positioning the machine than others – practice no doubt makes perfect. (That is the aspect of the treatment that worries me, in fact; I'm always a bit nervous about things that haven't been tested for twenty years or more and I do rather wish it had been going for a lot longer! I do feel rather brave, a bit of a pioneer, for trying it out...)

'Each eye takes about twenty minutes, so the whole process eats up forty minutes from my day, and initially, it had to be done every other day for ten treatments. That could be quite hard for people to schedule into a busy lifestyle. After about 10 days, I noticed that the skin had begun to look fresher and more vibrant in the eye area. I wouldn't say that my fine lines and wrinkles were any shallower, but overall the tone of the skin was visibly and quite significantly improved. That improvement went on becoming more and more noticeable throughout the rest of the series of treatments and beyond, so that overall, my eye area looks much fresher – and, as a result, younger.

'I suppose my real frustration is that enlighten can only target the eye area. The zone around my mouth is in fact much more wrinkled, and I'd like a similar treatment there, too. The other downside is the cost: it's expensive. But overall I guess I feel it was worth it – just.'

Let there be light: the cheats

Intense Pulsed Light therapies give quite dramatic results – so it's hard to replicate that with an at-home treatment. Certainly, there's no cream on the market which can deliver the age-reversing benefits of IPL – and if there was, it would be prescribed as a drug, not something you can pick up in your nearest marbled beauty hall. (The only thing that comes close is Retin-A, a prescription-only drug based on vitamin A.) However, there are some make-up products that you can use to cheat with which can reproduce some of the actions of the light therapies...

■ A whole new category of cosmetics has been invented in the last couple of years: 'skin brighteners'. These are mostly designed to be worn under make-up and feature reflective particles that really do create the illusion of 'glowing' skin. Those I'd thoroughly recommend include Prescriptives Vibrant (available as a lotion and a cream), Guerlain Divinora Liquid Radiance (which features tiny particles of gold, suspended in a gel), Lancôme Maquisuperbe, Ultima II Glowtion Moisture Cream SPF15 and BeneFit High Beam (see RESOURCES).

■ Just as light is being harnessed in the ultra-high-tech machines, the cosmetics industry has embraced light technology, too, to create products that 'bounce' light off the complexion, for a 'soft focus' effect that works to create the optical illusion of younger skin. The key is to look for the words 'light-diffusing' on the packaging or ask the consultant to recommend a product that has a light-diffusing effect. Applied over one of the skin brighteners I've just mentioned, your skin really should glow.

■ Regular exfoliation will help skintone and overall glow, so that your complexion looks naturally more vibrant and 'alive' – for the how-to on exfoliating skin healthily, rather than harshly, follow the steps on page 152.

■ For tricks to camouflage wrinkles, check out the cheats at the end of the chapters on BOTOX® – THE LINE TAMER and FILL 'EM UP – THE INJECTABLES. To disguise broken veins, see page 116.

CHAPTER 11

The beauty buzz – non-surgical facelifts

Beauty therapists have always claimed that facial muscles, as much as muscles in the body, need exercising and gentle stimulation. In the early days, facials were strictly hands-on treatments. Now, many salons employ electric devices to help buzz away the signs of ageing. Some, extensions of the passive exercise machines used for body toning, work on the principle that well-toned muscles return tautness to sagging contours – while others focus more on revving up the skin. Others claim to do both.

These machines, for the most part, have a medical heritage, being versions of a technology developed to treat athletes suffering from soft-tissue injury (such as whiplash or sprains), or to treat facial paralysis in Bell's Palsy patients. In non-surgical facelifts, the skin gets a muscle-stimulating blast of micro-currents – infinitesimal pulsating currents of electricity, tuned to mimic those which naturally take place at cellular level. It's usually done through probes, moved over the face by a beauty therapist or aesthetician to strengthen and tone the muscles. Muscles around the mouth, for instance, are shortened – so pulling up any deep furrows, while the 'corrugator' muscles (which create frown-lines) are lengthened. The bonus, meanwhile, is that the micro-stimulation of the skin gives circulation a boost – putting back some of the glow that ageing takes away.

The treatments vary from device to device: some use pads which stick to the face, while others are equipped with disk- or wand-shaped probes that are stroked over the skin. However it's distributed, the current – which, depending on the gizmo, can be so high as to make the facial muscles dance, so low it's imperceptible, or simply gives a faint tingling sensation to the skin – is ultimately claimed to give a 'lift' to the face, energise 'tired' cells and improve circulation. (Some companies also claim the treatments aid the penetration of lotions and potions.)

Many experts are sceptical about the possibility of plugging into electricity to erase the signs of ageing – especially since there are no scientific studies to validate the claims. But the main problem, in my experience, is that these treatments aren't very lifestyle-friendly. Most require an initial series of appointments, carefully timed to ensure a precise, prescribed amount of time elapses between treatments. If you've a busy diary prone to last-minute changes, this can play havoc with your treatment schedule and mean you don't get the intended benefit. Generally, a follow-up 'booster' treatment is also needed if you want to maintain the effects. (The gaps between these vary from brand to brand.)

For the nervous, though, these non-surgical facelift treatments may be an alternative to some of the more medically-based techniques I've outlined in the first half of this book. They're carried out by trained beauty therapists rather than doctors or nurses and the results, to be frank, are less dependent on the skills of the person who's giving you your non-surgical facelift than on the technology itself. In general, the worst reports I've come across are complaints that the treatment didn't live up to expectation (and so was a waste of money), and the most unpleasant side effect I've encountered is reports of a metallic taste in the mouth during treatment, by patients who have mercury fillings. There are generally no risks associated with these non-surgical facelift treatments, and recovery is instant. In fact, you should look better than when you walked through the salon door.

What are the downsides? These treatments have been in medical use for some twenty years or so, long before the beauty world embraced them for face enhancement. There are no known adverse effects – although anyone concerned with electromagnetic radiation (also emitted by mobile telephones, bedside clocks, radio masts and almost every electrical device you can name) would probably give non-surgical facelifts a wide berth. But the whole field of electromagnetic radiation is as yet so new and uncharted that any link between specific electrical devices and/or treatments and human health would probably take years to establish. As with everything in life, we have to think – and decide the risk/benefit ratio for ourselves.

As for suitability, for the most part, electrotherapy treatments are contra-indicated for people with pacemakers, epilepsy, active skin diseases, metal pins or plates in the immediate area or recent scar tissue. They should also be avoided by pregnant women. You should, as a matter of course, be asked for a full medical history before going ahead with a course of treatments.

I certainly have friends who swear by non-surgical facelift-type treatments – especially if they have a special occasion coming up (like a wedding or a very important date or job interview), and, in particular, just before having their photo taken professionally. When most of us need all the help we can get...

Dibitron M Time Machine

The low-down Dibitron is designed to substitute the human touch by a skilled and tireless massage therapist with incredibly strong fingers! The equipment consists of a spaceman-like helmet, inside which are a series of pads which are placed at the back of the neck, on the cervical vertebrae, the trapezius muscle at the front, and on the chin, jaw, cheeks and forehead. Controlled by an electronic micro-processor, these expand and contract within the mask, reproducing the effects of a hands-on massage.

Suitable for
Any type of skin, even acne-prone skins (who can also be helped by the stimulation offered by the machine) and those affected by couperose (severe broken veins), usually linked with skin sensitivity.

Not suitable for
Claustrophobes and those with neck problems/whiplash etc.

Upkeep
An initial course consists of ten treatments carried out a week apart, followed by twice-yearly treatments as maintenance

How much it costs
£45–65 per treatment, depending on the skincare products used.

CASE STUDY   **'I had Dibitron treatments'**

– DEBORAH, 44

'I'm not a believer in cosmetic surgery – but I think it's fine to be "unnaturally natural", using every other trick in the book short of the knife. I started having BOTOX® about two years ago – as an actress, my face is my fortune – and I've ended up having it done around every three months, to maintain the results. But since I had my first Dibitron treatment five months ago, I haven't needed the BOTOX® again. (To be honest, I didn't even really mean to have BOTOX®; I went to Dr Sebagh, in London, for a facial and his therapist said, "You should try this" – so I did. I was amazed at how shiny and flat it made my face; I don't think I had such a young forehead even when I was born! The minute it would wear off – after a couple of months, actually – I'd see what almost looked like a rash on my forehead, but in fact, it was the lines coming back...)

'A year or so ago I bumped into a girlfriend who looked fantastic and told me it was because of her Dibitron treatments, but it went in one ear and out the other. Then after my marriage broke up and I'd been having a hard time, she gave me a voucher for a Dibitron facial. At the salon I go to, the whole procedure lasts an hour and a half and the first hour uses lots of different masks, including DiBi and La Prairie, as well as special eye masks. Then the therapist puts a wet, gauze-y piece of fabric over the face before the Hannibal Lecter-like Dibitron mask itself is put on, on the front of the face and back of the neck, and screwed together. It's quite horrible-looking and made of metal, and inside are airbag-like attachments which get inflated during the treatment. By then, thanks to the preliminary facial, I'm very relaxed – which is just as well because it could be quite claustrophobic for some people; I have one friend who has it done and I have to go along and hold her hand while she's having the treatment because it makes her nervous – though she still thinks it's worth it.

'Then the machine starts pulsating and it feels like all your fillings are going to shake out – it's like a toning table for the face and you really feel it giving your muscles a workout, but it's nothing like CACI (which I've also had, and did nothing for me); with this, you really feel your face moving. I was worried about what would happen if I sneezed, but apparently the machine cuts off if that happens. It lasts for half an hour, and I find it so relaxing that now I'm like Pavlov's dog: the minute the machine's switched on, I'm asleep. At the salon I go to, they paint my toenails and fingernails while it's happening. At the end, you look in the mirror and see instantly that your face is tighter. From now on, I should only need twice-yearly treatments to keep up the good work, but initially, it does need a commitment to ensure the programme of weekly treatments is followed religiously.

'The glow from the treatments means that I now no longer need to wear make-up or even tinted moisturiser – just a tiny bit of blusher and lipstick. The lines that run from my nose to lips have virtually disappeared, over ten treatments, and people are always coming up to me and telling me how great I look. That hadn't happened for years!'

CACI Quantum

The low-down CACI Quantum is the newest, most high-tech version of the CACI system, which has over twenty years of medical research behind it and is the original non-surgical face-and-body lifting treatment, initially used to treat victims of strokes and facial palsy. The CACI Quantum is a versatile machine that can be used to create a tailor-made programme for your skin. (The machine can also be set to treat cellulite, enhance the bust and diminish stretch marks.) The programme includes a 'Lymph Drainage' mode, which works on lymph drainage points in the face and neck to drain excess fluid and remove puffiness, as well as a 'Micro-Mode', which can help to de-bag eyes and (again) enhance lymphatic drainage. A micro-current, conducted through cotton-tipped probes – or adhesive pads, applied to specific points in the face – perks up sagging facial muscles and helps smooth fine lines for a temporary 'lifting' effect. (The machine is linked to a cardiac monitor so that it works in rhythm with your heartbeat.) Some devotees insist, however, that if the initial treatment schedule is stuck to religiously, this 'lifting' effect is much more permanent; the idea is that the muscles can be 're-educated' to become toned again. If you have fillings, meanwhile, you're likely to have a metallic taste in your mouth.

Suitable for Generally aged and sagging skin, sun-damaged and dry, dehydrated skin, acne scarring, problematic oily skins.

Not suitable for The system works more effectively on older skins, to soften lines and wrinkles – those with younger-looking skin may not see significant results.

Upkeep Initially, between ten and fifteen treatments (depending on your skin condition and muscle tone, rather than your passport age!), with three treatments in the first week, followed by two treatments a week after that. Follow-up treatments every four to six weeks are recommended to maintain the benefits.

How much it costs From £45 per session.

CASE STUDY   **'I had CACI Quantum treatments'**

– DERRY, 44

'I was in my late thirties when I started to have CACI treatments, using an earlier version of the Quantum technology. I'd noticed that my jaw had started to "go" and gravity had generally started to kick in, and I'd started to see the odd fine line emerging; I'd fallen into the trap of having sunbeds back when everyone thought they were harmless, and am now paying the price. So I read about CACI in a magazine and thought it might be the solution.

'I was a bit nervous, but then someone gave me ten treatments as a generous birthday present. I was booked in for ten treatments – the prescribed series: four in the first week, a couple the next week, then once a week and ultimately every three weeks. (I was told if I messed up the schedule and missed appointments, I'd be back at square one, which is quite an incentive to keep going.) At the first session, the therapist did just half the face and got me to look in the mirror – and that was me, hooked. On the side that had been treated, the lines were definitely softened and my face looked visibly "lifted".

'Initially, my make-up is removed – not that I wear much, just enough to get around in public; I don't pile it on. Then a firming gel is applied around the jaw and eye area and the therapist places the probes on the skin. They're like little metal prongs with Q-Tip-like cotton ends. It's exactly like having a massage, but with a gizmo rather than someone's fingers. All of the movements are in an upwards direction – you feel as if your face is being gently pulled upwards, starting at the jaw and ending above the eyes. You can almost feel the eyes opening as the treatment progresses; after about ten to fifteen minutes, there's a definite "facelift" sensation and it all just feels tighter and firmer. There's absolutely no doubt that something's going on. Initially, I felt a little buzzing but by the second session I'd got used to the sensation and now I don't have any sense at all that there's electricity involved. I was warned that I might have a metallic taste in my mouth because of an interaction between the saliva and mercury fillings, but I don't have many fillings and have never experienced that.

'After each treatment, as well as the tightening and firming, the skin looks more translucent and fresh. For a few days afterwards, I really notice that my make-up goes on beautifully, because my skin's so smooth. But while the CACI Quantum does cleanse deeply and help circulation, it's really the noticable firming benefits that keep me going back for more.

'Because I saw results immediately, that incentivised me to stick to the treatment plan; although it was initially time-consuming, it was worth it. I was lucky; the salon I go to stays open late so I was able to go after work and I used to look forward to lying down and chilling out for an hour. Now, I try to go once a week – or if I have a special occasion coming up like a wedding – and if I try to penny-pinch and stretch the gap to six weeks between treatments, I really notice the difference and friends start to say, "Are you OK? You look a bit tired…" It's not so much that the face physically drops, but that freshness isn't there. I've had children and can't expect to defy nature, really, but I could pass for mid-to-late thirties. I certainly feel happy telling people

I'm forty-four – which I might not if I didn't look good for my age! I do have to budget for it, though. Now I have a good relationship with the salon and they tell me if there are special offers on a series of treatments, so I can get the best price.

'My mother says, "I wish I'd had this in my day..." She's had a couple of treatments and although her face looks more vibrant, it hasn't had the facelifting effect on her that I feel it has on me. With luck, by starting early, I'll be able to fend off surgery this way.'

ERP Face Magic™

The low-down ERP Face Magic™ is short for Electroridopuncture Face Magic, a treatment that involves the insertion of fine electrodes just underneath the skin, delivering a faradic-type current directly into dermis and sub-dermal tissues, so stimulating collagen production and boosting muscle tone. Seven electrodes are placed on each side of the face; there's also a specific, needle-type electrode with a different current which can be applied to individual lines and wrinkles or lips for a spot-targeted treatment. To address concerns about infection from needles, according to Dr Elisabeth Dancey (who introduced ERP Face Magic™ in the UK), 'Everyone has their own needles which are labelled and checked with the patient before each use.' (Practitoners of ERP Face Magic™ must be fully trained and accredited by Dr Dancey, who, as she puts it, 'reinvented the technique'; it's done by doctors, nurses and aestheticians. Dr Dancey says that the aestheticians are often particularly talented 'because they're so good with their hands'.)

Suitable for Faces with sagging and loss of tone, as well as fine lines, wrinkles and dull skin. According to Dr Dancey, 'The most important benefit of ERP Face Magic™ is that it addresses the problem of muscle tone. It maintains muscle tone in younger faces and restores lost tone in the older face. It also has a direct effect on the production of new, healthy collagen and elastin.' As Dr Dancey puts it, 'Consider it like a trip to the face gym.'

Not suitable for Anyone with a very low pain threshold (although in extremis, local anaesthetic – in the form of topical anaesthetic – may be applied). It's described as 'slightly uncomfortable', but one colleague of mine discontinued her series of treatments on the third visit, because, as she put it, 'It was simply excruciating.' Others, however, experience almost no discomfort. (NB Some women become more sensitive to pain while suffering from PMS or while having a period, so you may want to schedule your treatments accordingly.)

Recovery time Most women are able to go back to work/out to lunch/whatever immediately afterwards, although one patient I spoke to – who admittedly bruises easily – described herself as 'black and blue' after the treatment.

The risks Anyone allergic to nickel may have a minor allergic reaction to the needle, developing a mosquito-bite-like lump. In these cases, Dr Dancey recommends taking an anti-histamine tablet on the day of subsequent treatments. But she has also found that in those patients who start out allergic to the needle, ongoing treatments may have a stabilising effect on the immune system, so that the body stops reacting to the nickel of its own accord.

Upkeep For optimum benefits, twelve to fifteen weekly sessions should be followed with a maintenance regime of one session every six to eight weeks, although there's no limit to the number of sessions you can have.

How much it costs From £80 per session.

CASE STUDY   'I had Face Magic'

– CLARE, 59

'My problem is straightforward: old age. I am sixty next year and frankly, after a while, your skin begins to look dead. I don't have much sun damage – working in an office has kept me out of the sun, mostly – but I do have some lines around my chin which I blame on the dentist. (I think they may be related to dental X-rays, although I've no proof; I just can't think of another explanation.) As I've grown older, I've lost fat from my face, too. The temptation is to cover up the face with more and more make-up – but that's actually much more ageing.

'I tried collagen and couldn't stomach the pain, so I was a little nervous about Face Magic; I warned that I might scream the place down. Small needles are placed superficially in the skin, a little like acupuncture, and linked up to a small electrical current. (I was incredibly anxious the first time, convinced I was going to fry to death – but I didn't.) There's never been any pain from the needles – except once, when I was a bit tense, and she put a needle in my forehead; I said it hurt – and the needle was moved. When the needles are in place, you're given a metal bar to hold – that completes the electrical circuit, and the current passes through the needles in a kind of wave pattern, tingling as it goes; the tingling is stronger around the lips, but never crosses over into being painful. Altogether, the treatment lasts around half an hour; immediately afterwards, I might find I'm a little red and blotchy around the needle points, but by the time I've driven home ten minutes later, that's disappeared.

'I'm now so relaxed during treatments that I fall asleep; I find the current strangely comforting. My skin texture has improved immeasurably and the fine lines and wrinkles are much less visible, especially around my upper lip where the collagen has been shocked into rebuilding itself, plumping out the feathery lines. I've had a complete course of Face Magic, and now go back once a month for maintenance. I've also had a little BOTOX® in my forehead, with great

results; I don't look surprised or unnatural, and I can move my
eyebrows normally, so I'm pleased with that, too.

'Most people certainly don't think I'm the age I am. At nearly sixty,
you can't ask better than that, can you?'

Futur-Tec

The low-down This is a very versatile treatment – in fact, it's quite
hard to categorise because of its 'smorgasbord' approach: it uses
ultrasound to peel and cleanse, micro-current to soften lines and
wrinkles, vacuum to firm and enhance skintone – and laser (so Futur-
Tec's information sheet says), to encourage the natural production of
fibroblast cells, collagen and elastin. (However, when I checked on
this with Futur-Tec, they explained that the wavelengths of laser
light used by the Futur-Tec machine are not associated with any form
of skin damage.) After analysing your individual skin woes, the
therapist will prescribe a personalised treatment which may
incorporate different applications and uses of the Futur-Tec machine.
The 'Ultrasound Wave Actuator' emits non-abrasive ultrasonic
vibrations into the skin, to exfoliate dead cells, blackheads, make-up
residue etc; at the same time, bacteria will be sterilised, circulation
stimulated and cell turnover gently boosted. The 'Vaculase Actuator'
is a combined vacuum laser system that stimulates the lymphatic
system and local metabolism (putting back skin's 'glow') and directly
stimulating collagen and elastin (resulting in a selective 'lifting
action' on wrinkles). The 'Microlase Wrinkle Comb' combines laser
and electro-stimulation to improve skin regeneration and improve
elasticity, while the 'Laserstim Actuator' delivers a low-energy light
stimulus to improve skin oxygenation, 'unblock' the body's electrical
pathways and give the body's own healing system a helping hand.
Just to complicate matters further, there are special products for use
with each phase of the treatment – a Pre-Peeling solution for use with

the ultrasound phase, Healing Gel (used if the treatment is to combat acne or hyperpigmentation), Liquid Gold (a blend of natural oils for use with the Vaculase Actuator) and a Moisturising Gel; the idea is that when used in tandem with the treatment, their effectiveness is turbo-charged. Phew. (But happily, a trained therapist will work out which of these combinations you need…)

Suitable for On the face, Futur-Tec can be used to treat deep lines, wrinkles, stretch marks, acne, blemishes and hyperpigmentation.

Not suitable for Broken skin or open acne.

Recovery time You can face the world immediately afterwards.

Upkeep Initially, a course of ten, then, once a month.

How much it costs From £45 per session.

CASE STUDY
'I had Futur-Tec'

– ALISON, 37

'Even though I've lived in the sun, I have always protected my skin and don't feel I have a lot of lines. But my skin was very dry and sensitive – and as a result, had a crêpiness and redness that's associated with ageing skin, which made me look old. (I also flush easily after exercise or when I'm embarrassed and am generally a bit of a 'pink' person.) I'm definitely interested in anything that keeps ageing at bay but has minimal risks. I read about Futur-Tec in a newspaper, and saw in a subsequent ad that a salon near me had the equipment. I've had a few facials, in the past, but nothing very high-tech.

'At the initial consultation, I filled in a client form and as I lay on the couch, the therapist asked what I'd like to get from the treatment and

what my skin worries were. I explained about the dryness and
sensitivity. The Futur-Tec machine is big and modern, all silver and
whiz-bang high-tech. It's on wheels so it can be moved around if
necessary during the treatment, and on me, they used all the phases
except the one for acne, which isn't one of my skin worries.

'To start with, the beauty therapist does a normal cleanse, then the
laser phase, which is meant to be healing. There's no heat or pain at
all. This is followed by the peeling phase, with a special solution that
feels quite wet, cooling but pleasant on the skin. (And although I have
very "touchy" skin, I've never reacted to any of the products used in
the facial.) Then comes the "combing" phase which is the only one
with any discomfort; a pronged comb works on the wrinkles and lines,
including those around the eyes – and it's borderline painful, prickling
as it moves over the face.

'Immediately afterwards, I am a little red but this subsides. I
wouldn't say that I looked in the mirror after my first treatment and felt
like my face was instantly lifted, but it looked and felt smoother and
firmer. Each time I have had the treatment, I have felt that my skin
stays better for longer. Initially I had a series of six treatments, once a
week, and now I go once a month; I treat it as my regular facial.

'The treatment itself is very relaxing – once you get used to the
noises and learn to filter them out; the machine beeps, the ultrasound
makes it vibrate; the pitch constantly changes. The noises might be
quite unsettling for a nervous person, but I don't have a problem with
them and have learned to focus on the background music. In fact, after
a while, the beeping becomes quite hypnotic and I drift off.

'As the treatments have gone on, my characteristic redness has
really disappeared; now, I only flush if I exercise, rather than in daily
life. My skin is much less dry and not papery at all – in fact, it looks
glowing and dewy. Normal, in fact. I know it must be the facials
because I haven't changed anything else in my skin regime. (Although
having the facials has made me more conscious about bad habits;
paying all this money for facials, I wouldn't dare to fall into bed with

my make-up on, now – which wasn't always the case!) I now actually get compliments on my skin – which is certainly something that never happened before. I am an accountant's assistant, not a lunching lady, and I wouldn't be splashing out this money if I couldn't see significant results.'

Non-surgical facelifts: the cheats

■ If these non-surgical facelifts are like toning tables for the face, then Eva Fraser's Facial Workout is the equivalent of pulling on your leotard and getting to the gym to tighten your muscles. Though it requires dedication, many women swear by Eva's facial workouts (for which, in her smooth-faced seventies, Eva is her own best advertisement). For details of how to get hold of Eva Fraser's tapes, videos and books (or book in for one-on-one sessions to learn the technique face-to-facialist), see RESOURCES. Meanwhile, I asked Eva to share here a couple of her exercises for turning back the clock by firming the cheekbones...

UPPER CHEEK LIFT – BASIC EXERCISE 1

1 Place side of index fingers along laugh lines.

2 Now lift all four muscles upwards using your muscles.

3 Make very small lifting movements; do six lifts altogether, so that your muscle-lifting action moves your fingers.

4 Hold for a count of six.

5 Return slowly in six movements.

6 Repeat once more. KEEP EYES RELAXED.

UPPER CHEEK LIFT – BASIC EXERCISE 2

1 Touch face with middle fingers just under the outside of the eye.

2 Keep your back teeth lightly together, lips apart as you smile upwards towards your temples in six slow movements. Feel the muscle lift each time.

3 Hold for a count of six.
4 Return slowly in six movements.
5 Repeat once more. DO NOT SQUINT.

■ 'Firming' and 'lifting' are two of the beauty world's hottest buzzwords right now, as baby boomers hit crunch-time. (I recently flicked through a magazine targeted at women of forty-plus, and the first seven ads were for cosmetics that featured the word 'lift' in the name.) These creams can't possibly deliver the instant effect of a non-surgical facelift – but used over time, they may slightly enhance facial firmness. I've had particularly good reports about Lancôme Rénergie Contour Lift, Givenchy Firm Profile and the Clarins Extra Firming Range; these skin treats are designed to show benefits with regular use over anything from a fortnight to a month or more.

■ At a pinch, whipped egg white, applied to the face, has an astonishing tightening effect; in the old days, Hollywood stars would allegedly slather this on their faces and then apply make-up over the top, to create the illusion of smooth, line-free skin. (Do not experiment immediately before an important event; this is a technique for which practice makes perfect.)

■ A product called No Lines, also by Victoria Vogue (see RESOURCES), works in roughly the same way as the whipped egg white: you place a drop of this 'tautening solution' on the end of your finger or cotton swab and apply directly to fine lines and puffy areas. Smooth it outwards and away from lines in a feathering motion, until any excess is removed – and then don't touch. Allow to dry for three to five minutes. (If a white film forms after drying, moisten your fingertips with warm water and blend into the skin.) You can then apply make-up over the top.

■ As long as you're not expecting anyone to run their fingers
through your hair or get too up-close-and-personal, you could
resort to the 'Traynor Lift', as sometimes used by (fading)
actresses of stage, screen and DVD to give a more youthful look
to the face. It's actually a kit containing surgical tape which is
attached to two pieces of elastic, which can be applied to the
skin in several different zones to pull the face upwards and
backwards when the pieces of elastic is secured behind the head.
(Literally recreating the effect if you do the same thing with your
fingers, in front of the mirror.) Make-up can be applied over the
top. But be warned, this doesn't bear too-close scrutiny and
needs plenty of hair – in a style that partly covers the face – to
disguise both the elastic and the spots where the tapes are stuck
to the face.

CHAPTER 12

The überfacials

Skincare salons have always offered a range of services that soothed the spirit while providing a kind of spring-clean for the skin. But now their menus are loaded with facial treatments that also promote rejuvenation. Nobody's claiming that these will have as dramatic an effect as a shot of BOTOX®, a syringe-ful of collagen or a blast with an NLite™ laser – but for women who don't want to go down that route, they can offer definite (if fairly short-lived) skin benefits.

There are hundreds – if not thousands – of anti-ageing facials out there; I could have written an entire book on those alone. But in this section, I've narrowed them down to some 'überfacials': cosmetic treatments which, in my experience (and that of dozens women I've spoken to), offer real turn-back-the-clock benefits, making them ideal before a special occasion, or as part of your general anti-ageing strategy. They go way beyond the cleanse, tone and moisturise category. (In fact, for the acupuncture facial I mention, there's no pampering element at all. But boy, are the results effective; if necessary, I'll insist on being wheeled to see my facial acupuncturist in my bath chair.)

Nobody's really promising these are much more than temporary 'quick fixes'. But personally, I'm a great believer in regular facials for stimulating facial circulation and getting rid of general skin dinginess. Recovery time is zero: you should definitely expect to look better immediately afterwards – and if not, you'll want to know why! The only real risk attached to some of them is 'skin overload'; if you have particularly sensitive skin, it's possible that you could react to one or more of the ingredients in the products used in the multi-step treatments, setting off a chain-reaction when you encounter that ingredient in future. If you have sensitive skin, be sure to communicate this to the therapist before your treatment. You should, in any case, be asked for a full lifestyle history that will include some medical details. My advice, as always, is to be honest, and not to play down any medical problems or niggles you have just because you want the treatment to go ahead.

My one last tip? If a beauty therapist tries to sell you an entire new range of skincare 'to continue the improvements at home', don't fall for it – unless you're shopping for new skincare anyway. There's no evidence of synergistic benefits offered by using one specific skincare line while excluding all others. Take it from me – and they'll kill me for saying this – it's just marketing hype.

Acupuncture facial

(NB This should not be confused with ERP Face Magic™, which, although it uses needles, is quite different. For details of Face Magic, see page 181).

The low-down Facial acupuncture is carried out by trained acupuncturists – a cosmetic application of traditional Oriental acupuncture techniques. Although some acupuncturists also have a conventional Western medical training, many don't; decide if that's important for you, and if it is, you may like to reassure yourself by establishing your practitioner's background and qualifications before opting for treatment. There is no one system for facial acupuncture, because most facial acupuncturists develop their own technique, which may also include massage (see the case history that follows). By inserting acupuncture needles into the body's energy channels, or 'meridians', skin functions can be improved, restoring glow – or combating acne; devotees report that it's extremely good for 'tired' faces and can also have an effect on reducing frown-lines and giving a general 'lift'. (In fact, because of acupuncture's 'whole-body' approach, the therapist is working on all the body's organs – not just the visible organ, our skin, even when ministering to the needs of the face.) Before you start, however, the acupuncturist will usually take a full medical history and use various forms of diagnosis to establish your overall health. (The complexion is just one clue.) C.Y. Yan, a New York-based doctor of traditional Oriental medicine, uses four kinds of analysis to reach her diagnosis: 'First is the sound of the voice over the phone. Second is how you look, how you carry yourself when you walk in. Third is how you smell – you'd be surprised what I can smell! – and fourth is the case history.' The practitioner will take your 'pulses' – three on each wrist, only one of which is listened to in Western medicine, and may ask you to stick out your tongue for examination. From this, the practitioner may be able to pin-point with astonishing accuracy personal details like the fact you skipped lunch today or that you're ovulating! Then, while you recline on the couch, needles will be inserted – usually painlessly (although there may be a twinge) – in different areas of the body, as well as the face. (As an example, some might be placed in the arms and legs, one on the top of the head, between the eyebrows, the chin, laugh-lines.) The session may finish with facial massage – or not. If you're unsure what to expect, ask. Facial acupuncture treats the whole body – not just the complexion, which is why patients often report that their mind feels sharper and they have more energy after a treatment. (In fact, I believe anyone considering any form of treatment in this book would be wise to embrace a holistic approach to rejuvenation, working on overall wellbeing, not just the facial manifestation of ageing...)

Suitable for Skin problems such as acne and allergies, as well as tired faces that have lost their youthful 'glow'.

Not suitable for Needle phobics.

Recovery time Zero. (Although you may just feel a little woozy or light-headed afterwards; alternatively, you may feel like doing energetic cartwheels. This varies from patient-to-patient and sometimes, treatment-to-treatment).

The risks You need to be sure that the needles the acupuncturist uses are clean and specific to you, because of the concerns about infection with HIV, hepatitis or other blood-borne infections. Most acupuncturists now use fresh needles as a matter of course for each new patient, but if you're in any way concerned, ask for reassurance.

Upkeep As often as you like. (Some patients go weekly, others monthly – and others just twice a year; the changeover of seasons – from winter to spring, summer to autumn – are good times.)

How much it costs From £55 per facial.

CASE STUDY   **'I had an acupuncture facial'**

– JOANNA, 45

'I have had acupuncture before, for minor health problems like cystitis (on which it had near-miraculous results), so I knew what to expect from this treatment. I avoid the sun like the plague and have very few lines and wrinkles – I often get a lot of compliments for my skin – but I work very hard and often look quite tired and stressed. I wanted something that would "put back the glow", and read about acupuncture facial in a magazine.

'Yuki Umeguchi – who I believe has also treated Madonna and Courtney Love, among others – took a full medical history before she started the facial, and also placed her fingers on my wrist to check my "pulses". (In Oriental medicine, we have more than one pulse.) I had to poke out my tongue and show her.

'She explained that our faces reflect our inner health and wellbeing, so it's not enough to slap on creams and lotions and hope that's enough. After our ten-minute consultation, she asked me to remove my tights, trousers and top and to lie down on the couch under a warm blanket. I was expecting needles only in the face – after all, this was a facial – and so I was a bit surprised when she placed them between my toes, in my hand and wrist, my breastbone and even the top of my head. There was absolutely no pain when the needles went in – a slight twinge, that's all, except for the needle in the top of the head which hurt a lot. She also placed needles around my face: between my brows, my cheeks… Again, there was zero pain, which I was surprised by. After a few minutes, she removed the needles from my face and began massaging it, leaving the needles in the rest of my body. Actually, the motions are more like subtle pushing and pulling, and pressure – for instance, under the cheekbones – than actual soothing massage. She continued with these movements for around fifteen minutes, before removing the needles from elsewhere – and handed me a mirror. I was truly astonished; my face looked firmer, rosier and much more youthful. In fact, I had that "rested" look that I usually only get after a good holiday! I would say that I looked five years younger, easy. For a week or two after the treatment, everyone was asking if I'd been away.

'I can't say the results are permanent, but they are so impressive that I now have these treatments at least once a month, and more if I have an important occasion or am having my photograph taken. It's much, much more than a facial, though – more like an overall tune-up, with knock-on benefits for my whole health and wellbeing. I once went along feeling like I'd been fighting a cold and wishing it would just happen, so my body could deal with it. Yuki placed two needles either side of my nose and within ten minutes, my nose had started streaming and she had to hold a tissue to it, because I was pinned to the couch like Gulliver! It just emphasised to me how incredibly powerful these treatments are. In actual fact, I'm a beauty editor by profession; I get to try every treatment under the sun for free. But the one I choose to pay for, and to have in preference to all the free treatments I could have, is this acupuncture facial. I think that says it all.'

Endolite Lift 6

The low-down This is a new 'face-shaping' machine from Endermologie®, whose body treatment device has been approved by the US Food and Drug Administration for the treatment of cellulite. Endermologie® uses a unique rolling and sucking action to work on cellulite and body contouring, reduction of scar tissue and the reduction of lactic acid build-up in athletes. The new Endolite Lift 6 targets facial muscles only, using what's known as 'the Jacquet technique': Parisian Dr Jacquet (of the Sainte-Antoine Hospital in Paris) discovered that by manipulating the delicate facial connective tissues with his fingers – using a gentle pinching action – he could stimulate the skin, tangibly reducing lines and wrinkles. This Lift 6 is a mechanised version of that massage, using a pulsed suction device which moves across the skin in sliding, lifting and spiral movements to decongest and oxygenate the skin, improving elasticity and firmness, leaving the face looking 'lifted'.

Suitable for All kinds of tired-looking and ageing faces.

Not suitable for Skins with active acne.

Upkeep An initial course of twelve sessions, twice a week, is recommended; the treatments last for thirty-five minutes, with monthly treatments for maintenance.

How much it costs Approximately £35–£50 per treatment, depending on the salon.

CASE STUDY   'I had Endolite 6'

— HANIA, 46

'One day I just woke up and realised I was losing my looks. My skin's not too bad, I use good cosmetics (La Prairie), I don't have too many wrinkles – but I had lost that glow. I've always been interested in alternatives to the knife because surgery scares me, so I really liked the sound of Endolite when my facialist told me about it.

'It starts with a cleanse, and then the treatment itself is very relaxing – a good feeling, like a stimulating facial massage. I'm a real coward and was pleased to discover there's no discomfort whatsoever. It feels as if someone is massaging you manually – but in fact, it's a machine being used. The equipment has three different "head" attachments. One is to detoxify, one is for the actual massage and the last one is what I call "the wrinkle eater"; it feels as if it's picking up dust from your skin, like a baby Hoover. The sensation is as if you were pinching your own skin. These are used in sequence, while you lie there with your eyes shut. The finale is a beautiful mask – and then (because the salon I go to uses La Prairie), I request one of their serum ampoules to be massaged into my skin. The skin seems to absorb whatever "goodies" are put on it at this point particularly well, so that it looks dewy and very well-moisturised.

'I am always running right, left and centre but I fall asleep every time during these treatments because they're sublimely relaxing. So far, I've had about fifteen to twenty treatments – three times a week in the first week, twice a week from the second week onwards until the end of the course; now, I go for maintenance once a month. There's been a slight improvement in the fine lines and wrinkles, but what I really noticed from the very first treatment is that I've got my youthful glow back again. I think one has to be a bit philosophical about wrinkles – they're inescapable – but what really makes you look old is a tired complexion; that's what people notice. Mine now looks fresh and vibrant like it used to, and I couldn't be more pleased.'

Environ Ionzyme facial

(NB Although there are a million facials out there, I've included this one because it incorporates electrical pulses and ultrasound to boost the penetration of anti-ageing treatments by, so the manufacturers claim, 'up to 4000 per cent'. Certainly, the before-and-after pictures are exceptional.)

The low-down This facial uses the Environ range of cosmetics, developed by South African Dr Des Fernandes. During treatment, the Ionzyme machine uses a pulsed galvanic (electrical) current and waves of sound (ultrasound) 'to help penetration of ingredients including vitamins A, C, E and betacarotene between the cells of the skin's horny layer' (according to Environ). After cleansing and toning, a mild lactic acid is applied and the skin covered with a damp gauze – including eyelids, nose and lips – over which a conductive gel is painted. 'Crocodile clips' are attached to the edge of the gauze, via which the current is conducted for twenty minutes. This is followed by a hydrating massage with an oil rich in vitamins A and E, two masks, and a second gauze treatment – this time, to help penetration of a serum and gel which are rich in antioxidants and/or (in the case of pigmented, scarred or sun-damaged skin) salicylic acid. During this second gauze treatment, holes may be cut in the gauze to treat specific problem areas for five minutes each, using the ultrasound probe.

Suitable for Photo-aged, pigmented, acne- or eczema-prone skin; the Ionzyme Facial is particularly effective on problem areas such as the eyes, neck or upper lip, working to minimise fine lines, wrinkles and crêpiness.

Not suitable for Women with sensitivity to alpha-hydroxy 'fruit acids' (aka AHAs). In fact, I'd suggest that women with sensitive skin probably steer clear of this facial, because of its high level of active ingredients – or ask for a 'patch test' in which the different products used in the facial are applied to a sensitive zone of the body (e.g. behind the ear or on the inner arm), while they wait to see if any redness, soreness or itchiness emerges.

Upkeep Initially, twelve treatments once or twice weekly are recommended, followed by a once-a-month maintenance schedule. (NB The dramatic results in the woman featured in the literature – whose neck literally looks like it had been lifted – had twenty-four twice-weekly treatments, the full benefits of which were still apparent six months after the course had finished. This could prove pretty expensive.)

How much it costs Around £60 for a full, ninety-minute facial.

CASE STUDY   'I have Environ vitamin facials'

– KATE, 44

'I could see time creeping onwards on my face, and felt it was time for action. My skin was in reasonable condition, but not great, and the areas I was most concerned about were the fine lines around the mouth and big pores around the central zone of my face. I'm not great about doing all the right things, like eating properly, not drinking and staying out of the sun, or knocking back three litres of water a day, so I have to do something to make up for that. A friend of mine who's South African raved about the Environ range of cosmetics, and said this facial was all the rage over there, so I decided to give it a go.

'Initially, a gel is placed on your face, which stings a bit. Then a gauze is laid over that, which calms the stinging down a bit, and metal clips attached to the gauze to conduct a light electrical current. At the same time, if you're worried about specific areas – pigmentation, for example, or areas of lines – another gel is applied to those and a metal probe is used to focus on treating that part of the face. I tend to ask the facialist to use the probe to focus on a different area each time, so that over the series of treatments, the whole face gets a mega-treatment. There's a slight tingling sensation from the current – a little like a C.A.C.I. facial – but nothing major.

'I wouldn't say it's the most pleasant experience in the world – not something you do for a bit of relaxation and a treat, but I feel the results speak for themselves. (There's certainly no chance of nodding off!) The first time – that facial lasted for an hour-and-a half, rather than the usual forty-five minutes – I could see a significant difference afterwards; my skin really did look more vibrant and "ironed out". Subsequently, there's been a slight glow afterwards – especially on areas that they've concentrated on, which look slightly smoother. But this isn't like C.A.C.I., where you can see the "lift" afterwards; with the Environ facial you have to have a bit of faith because the real improvements aren't seen for a while. At the same time, this is a much longer-lasting fix. After a few treatments – which initially I had twice a week, or once a week if I was really busy at work – my skin began to look much, much firmer and the overall skintone was much more even and fresher-looking. It feels more velvety, the fine lines aren't so deep, and the overall improvement is huge. Friends now comment that I look well even when I feel dog-tired – which can be a bit annoying when I want some sympathy! There are twelve treatments in a course – I buy a course at a time, because it's cheaper – and over the last year I've had two courses. I'm now into my third course which I use for occasional maintenance – say, once a month, or I'll book one specially if I've been out drinking. My skin never has that grey, tired look any more and I'm really impressed. This is something I plan to go on doing for a long, long time.'

Hydradermie

The low-down Guinot are calling this 'the new Cathiodermie for the 21st Century' – a 'new and improved' version of the classic (and well-loved) Cathiodermie treatment. During the facial, the appropriate Guinot cleanser and toner are applied. The therapist then massages using an exfoliating lotion, selecting a 'plant-based hydragel' appropriate to the skin's needs: aloe and shea butter for normal or dehydrated skin, malt extract for dry, mature skin, or chamomile and vitamin E for sensitive skin. Using special rollers that conduct a minute electrotherapy current, the skin is massaged to help the hydrogel penetrate deeper into the skin. A gauze soaked in lavender-rich emulsion is then smoothed over the skin, and high-frequency electrical current used to create an anti-bacterial effect on the skin's surface while boosting circulation. The final step is a plant-based, skintype-matched mask – with a dab of moisturiser and eye cream to send you back into the world again. Hydra Plus is a deluxe, ultra-pampering version of the Hydradermie treatment which offers specific benefits for the eyes, neck and décolletage, incorporating specialised serums for the eye and neck, and several spot-targeted masks. (NB Although Hydradermie uses an electrical micro-current, it can't really be categorised with the 'non-surgical facelifts'.)

Suitable for Aged, dehydrated and devitalised skins, in particular, should benefit from Hydradermie.

Not suitable for Epileptics and anyone with a metal plate in their head. Pregnant women are sometimes nervous about having

Hydradermie (formerly cathiodermie), but according to Guinot, there are no known risks.

Upkeep Initially, three treatments, once a week, then once every three weeks to a month, for maintenance.

How much it costs From £30.

CASE STUDY   'I swear by Hydradermie'

– MOLLY, 67

'I have been having Guinot Cathiodermie facials for twenty-five years and without wanting to blow my own trumpet, I don't look my age. I started them in my early forties, when I felt my skin needed extra help. I've had the facials once every six weeks since then and they're not only hugely enjoyable but I think have contributed to the firmness, smoothness and texture of my skin, which looks glowing and vibrant.

'Now I'm having the "new Cathiodermie" – Hydradermie – which I think is even better than the original. Before the facial starts you're lulled into a state of pure relaxation by a hand, arm and even ear massage. I really appreciate this bit because one of the worst things about getting older, for me, isn't my reflection in the mirror – it's the fact that when you're old, nobody touches you any more. This is followed by a deep cleanse and the multi-step facial. The unique element of the Hydradermie facial is the "roller" technique, using metallic probes that glide over the skin's surface. There's a tiny one – with a tip almost like a ball-bearing – to treat the area around the eyes, connected to an electrical current. With this ball-bearing roller, there's no tingling sensation – but the current is increased when the beauty therapist moves on to the larger probe. This is the shape and size of a small battery, and again is applied in massaging movements to the skin's surface, with a very smooth action. It tingles as it goes – but nothing uncomfortable; in fact, the cool feel of the metal is very soothing.

'There's the usual mask element to the facial, but what really makes a difference, I feel, are the rollers – which have a firming action. I always feel rejuvenated afterwards, as well as look it: my face is "lifted" as well as much healthier and alive-looking. The benefits last for about six weeks – and then I know it's time to book in again. But why I really like this more than the Cathiodermie is the hands-on element. Nothing beats that human touch.'

Rejuvenessence

The low-down Rejuvenessence is a facial massage technique that combines light movements with special toning strokes to regenerate the collagen and elastin tissue and stimulate the lymphatic, nervous and circulatory systems; like any facial massage, it will revive sluggish circulation, giving skin an instantly more healthy look. The massage also releases ingrained stresses and tensions in the muscles (ninety-one of them in the face, neck, skull and shoulders), allowing them to relax back into their natural positions; afterwards, the skin is smoother and looks plumper. According to Margareta Loughran, Rejuvenessence also 'detoxifies' the face. 'Toxicity reflects in the face in various ways and in different degrees. Bags under the eyes are the first sign; deep lines around the mouth and gray, ageing skin also mark a toxic face.' The treatment can also induce a trance-like state of relaxation. Initially – because Rejuvenessence takes a 'whole body' approach – you'll be asked to fill in a lifestyle and nutrition questionnaire. In the UK, only therapists who have been trained in Rejuvenessence by Margareta Loughran, based in London's Cheyne Walk (who introduced the technique from Scandinavia), are allowed to use the exact word 'Rejuvenessence' to describe their facials. However, some therapists have taken the movements and adapted them, giving their own, 'tweaked' version a different name. (In the US, a virtually identical technique goes by the name RejuvenEssence™.) Practitioners should already be trained as massage therapists, bodyworkers, aestheticians or cosmetologists, in order to have the required understanding of anatomy and physiology.

Suitable for Skin that is ageing, with lines and wrinkles, or has lost its 'bloom' and 'glow'. In addition, Rejuvenessence has been found helpful in treating chronic migraines, and has had some success at treating scar tissue, making it less obvious. As with an acupuncture facial, this pressure-point massage works 'holistically' – i.e. on the whole body; pressure points on the face correspond to other organs in the body, which should be (positively) stimulated by the massage, so that you don't just look better, but feel it.

Not suitable for Because this is (literally) a very 'hands-on' treatment, it may not be right if you don't like having your face constantly touched and 'played with', as this is the entire basis of the one-hour treatment. (Only one person I know didn't enjoy her treatments, though, saying she felt 'pawed and prodded'.)

Recovery time Zero, although I have had reports from friends who've suffered minor headaches after a Rejuvenessence treatment. (But then again, one Rejuvenessence devotee I spoke to described her treatment as 'like being on holiday'.)

Upkeep An initial series of six (usually one-hour) treatments is recommended, at intervals of one to two treatments per week; for maintenance, it's recommended that you have further massage sessions every two to three months.

How much it costs From approximately £25-60 per treatment, depending on the practitioner.

'I had Rejuvenessence'

– JO, 41

'About six months ago I'd been going through a tough time in my life and I really felt the strain was showing in my face. I looked at old photographs and felt it was time to do something – my skin wasn't bad, but my face (especially my jawline) had begun to sag and look puffy and jowly; I looked really stressed and my eyes were almost ghost-like, with dark circles.

'A friend told me about Rejuvenessence and it made me think it was time to focus on myself again to break out of that negative cycle; you feel bad, so you look bad, so you feel bad… I booked in with Margareta Loughran herself, though I wasn't sure what to expect – could the results be as good as a facelift? – but I was encouraged by the fact that I was able to have one treatment before I made up my mind whether to go for a course of five. (I hate it when beauty salons tell you you'll need eight sessions – and then demand money up front!) From the very first session, though, Rejuvenessence was quite amazing. In that session, she did the whole face – although in future sessions, individual problem areas (like the skin around the eyes or mouth) were spot-targeted; the strokes were incredibly light and soothing and I kept thinking, "this can't be doing any good." But halfway through I was handed a mirror to look at the difference between the two sides of my face – and it was really staggering; on one side my eye looked higher and "lifted", and the cheekbone was more prominent. Most importantly, my jaw looked firmer. At the end of the session I looked younger and fresher – no question, and certainly convinced enough to go back for the rest of the course, once a week.

'I'd had some CACI treatments in the past but they were nothing like as relaxing as this. Until I had Rejuvenessence, I was really unaware of how much tension I was carrying in my face – especially the jaw. Afterwards, it feels as if my face has much more freedom – as if it's somehow been "released". The movements are very small and contained – I feel the fingers connecting lightly with the muscle just underneath the skin. The benefits are definitely progressive: each time I can see an improvement. Importantly, I've become much more aware of the facial expressions I'm making – I have a tendency to frown, but because I now know that, I am increasingly able to stop myself. (Though I wouldn't say I'm completely cured, and at the end of a stressful day, I still find I'm scowling!) I think it's really important to gain that consciousness of our facial muscles; we concentrate so much on our skins – but not enough on what goes on underneath.

'It's incredibly relaxing. I've woken up with a snort, snoring, several times – which is embarrassing, but I'm sure therapists are used to it. I think it says a lot for the relaxing benefits of the treatment that it's possible to flop on a couch and switch off like that, in the middle of a busy day and a busy city. I think it's brilliant – a really interesting treatment that is hugely enjoyable. I now book a treatment when I want to look my best for something, or if I'm feeling particularly stressed-out and want that ironed from my face. Not only do I get the relaxation, but some tangible benefit that I can see. And that helps the positive spiral: you feel better, so you look better. It's all the facelift I feel I need, now.'

Überfacials: the cheats

At-home acupressure facial

Although you won't achieve the dramatic effects of an acupuncture facial – see page 191 – it is possible to get many of the turn-back-the-clock benefits of an Oriental treatment at home using pressure-point massage techniques in place of needles. (Do not try that at home!) These movements go back millennia; since ancient times, the Japanese and Chinese have worked on facial points to stimulate the skin by improving the flow of 'chi', the body's vital life force. Facial massage also works as an age-defier by reducing tension in the muscles, which can eventually etch lines in the face. And by increasing blood flow, this massage also delivers oxygen and essential nutrients to the skin, helping to drain away toxins from the cells. Your face should be firmer – and temporarily 'lifted'.

A simple, twelve-point pressure massage can help roll back the years – and put back the glow, eliminating tiredness and restoring lost 'glow'. Ideally, you should set aside twelve minutes for this facial acupressure-based massage. (If you want to time it, keep a clock with a second-hand where you can see it easily.) But even a few seconds spent on each acupressure point will make a difference to skin vibrancy. Why not incorporate it into your nightly cleansing regime: apply cleanser, massage facial acupressure points, then wash/remove cleanser as normal. Hey, presto: glowing skin...

Step–by–step facial acupressure

This can be done on bare or made-up skin, using a facial massage oil, or (as part of your nightly regime) with your regular cleanser. Using the middle finger of each hand, massage the points on either side of the face, which 'mirror' each other. (A few points are in the centre of the face; use the middle finger or either your right or left hand here.) If you've time, massage for up to one minute per pressure point. Otherwise (especially if you're doing this nightly), using this pressure point technique for just five or ten seconds on each point will help. The correct pressure doesn't skim over the surface; it moves the skin.

Remember: breathe deeply and rhythmically while enjoying this 'acupressure facelift'.

1 Locate the spot at the hairline that's directly above the centre of the eye. Massage using inward circles.

2 Move fingers down the face to halfway between eyebrows and hairline. Massage using inward circles.

3   This spot uses your thumbs: locate the spot on either side of the bridge of the nose, just below the brow-line. Push upwards, using pressure rather than circling technique. (NB This can hurt!)

4   At the outer tip of the eyebrows, massage with outward circles.

5   At the outside corner of the eyes, massage outwards.

6   On the top of the cheekbone, underneath the middle of the eye, circle outwards.

7   Now move the fingers down until they are in line with your nostrils, and massage using outward circles.

8   In the indentation that runs from the middle of your nose to your top lip, circle in a clockwise direction.

9   Locate the middle of your chin (where a 'dimple' would be), and again, massage in clockwise circles.

10 Using both fingers again, place fingers on the jawline either side of the chin. Circle outwards.

11 Move fingers outwards along the jaw to a point mid-way between jaw and the jaw hinge. Massage in outward circles.

12 Find the muscle just in front of the jaw hinge – there'll be a slight indentation. With the mouth resting open, circle towards the back of your head.

■ Two of the best at-home face masks I've ever found for delivering almost instant results are Liz Earle Brightening Treatment and Chanel Masque Lift Express, which – while not quite living up to Chanel's extravagant promise that it's 'as effective as a mini facelift in ten minutes' – does instantly get rid of a tired look, and leaves the face looking much less slack. (It contains yeast extract, hyaluronic acid, sweet white lupin and beech bud, which is known for a restructuring and smoothing effect. And, like all Chanel skin treats, it's bliss to use and looks sexy on the bathroom shelf.)

■ If skin's looking dingy, raid the fridge, where you should find the ingredients for this instant skin brightener:

Half an avocado
20 ml/1 tbsp tomato pulp
15 ml/1 tbsp lemon juice

Mash the skinned and pitted avocado with the other ingredients until you have a very smooth paste; spread over the face and neck (and hands, if you like) and leave for twenty minutes before washing off with warm water. Pat skin dry. For dehydrated skins, substitute 5 ml/1 tbsp of lemon juice and the same quantity of honey, leaving out the tomato pulp.

CHAPTER 13

Recovery mode

As I've explained, some people will react with redness and/or swelling to some of the procedures in this book. Most redness should subside within hours, if not a day or so. (If it doesn't, contact your doctor or salon for advice.) In the case of swelling, applying ice packs – available from pharmacies (and usually designed to tackle sports injuries) – should combat the problem.

Be sure to follow, to the letter, any instructions you're given, including staying away from heat and sunlight if advised. If you're prescribed any drugs by a doctor following your treatment, take them. If you're not freely given advice, then ask what kind of post-treatment TLC you should be giving your skin.

When it comes to make-up, however, you may want to switch – at least temporarily – to a range which is widely prescribed by cosmetic surgeons around the world for use after treatment. It was created by Jane Iredale, a British-born Broadway casting director/producer-turned-cosmetic-creator, who now lives in the US. This line is based on powdered mineral pigments, with not a single chemical in sight – so it's suitable for use even on broken skin, which would act as a 'vector' for the chemical ingredients in other products, introducing them directly into the bloodstream.

As a big fan of her range – for its naturalness and camouflage-power – I asked Jane for some specific advice.

■ 'Microdermabrasion and superficial or very superficial peels
are a piece of cake for mineral make-up,' says Jane. 'One light
layer is all you need. In fact, several of the major US peel
companies carry our minerals around with them to
demonstrate how effectively the residual redness can be
covered immediately after a treatment; they think this helps
sell their ranges. More importantly, the minerals have two
other benefits. The titanium dioxide and zinc oxide are anti-
inflammatories and help to calm the skin after any kind of
trauma. I have a client – a make-up artist – who peels his skin
so much that he applies the minerals immediately afterwards,
and goes to bed in them. He swears he gets less swelling and
redness this way. The zinc is also anti-microbial, so it will help
prevent infection.' Using a puff, apply Jane Iredale The
Skincare Make-up (which is a concealer, foundation, powder
and sunblock all-in-one) to the affected area. For lighter
coverage you could also use her Pure Pressed powder, whisking
away excess with a big, fluffy brush.

■ 'Any time the skin is peeled or micro-dermabraded,' explains
Jane, 'the stratum corneum – or top layer of skin – is removed.
This is actually the body's first layer of defence against the
damaging effects of the sun. Peeling the skin in this way leaves it
more vulnerable than ever. Mineral pigments replace the stratum
corneum with broad spectrum sun protection – that is, against
both UVA and UVB light – without the need for chemicals, and
so there's no risk of sensitising the skin, which has been
compromised by the treatment.' (And, she adds, 'It's important
to remember that though the redness may be very short-lived,
the loss of the stratum corneum is not, and the skin will
continue to be vulnerable until the natural process replaces it.
That replacement will take place more quickly, the younger you
are.')

■ 'Collagen can leave redness and bruising – and so can BOTOX®.
Again, the redness is easily covered with a yellow-based mineral
powder. For the bruises, I use Jane Iredale Circle/Delete #2,
which is a light and medium peach combination and contains
vitamin K. The darker peach really neutralises the blue of the
bruise. Then the minerals are 'stippled' over the concealer using
a camouflage brush for application. Circle/Delete can also be
used for any under-eye circles or other blemishes that appear on
the skin. The camouflage brush allows access to hard-to-reach
places like the corner of the eye, and doesn't drag the delicate
skin surrounding the eye.' (For more advice and info, I can
recommend you surf right over to www.janeiredale.com.)

Remember, too, that you're wasting your money on any kind of anti-
ageing treatment if you go on blithely exposing your skin to the sun.
You may even, potentially, risk turbo-charging damage to your skin
– in the case of treatments that work by removing the top layers of
skin – because it now has fewer layers of protection. If you want to
maintain your skin in its best condition for as long as possible,
s-t-r-e-t-c-h-i-n-g any benefits to the max, then you need to follow
the oft-repeated skin advice that beauty editors like me repeat on a
loop. Eat well, with plenty of wholegrains, vegetables and fruit. Keep
your face out of the sun, and protect it with an SPF15 when you're
out of doors. (Better still, wear a hat.) Drink two-and-a-half litres of
water a day. Exercise – both aerobically, and some form of stretching.
(Yoga will do more for your jawline than non-surgical facelift
machines ever can.) Get plenty of sleep. And try to stop worrying. At
least about your wrinkles, if not about global warming and world
peace...

Glossary

Ablation A process which vaporises the superficial layers of skin.

Acne Usually a chronic condition, with symptoms of inflamed breakouts or boil-like spots. (Occasional zits aren't usually classified as acne.)

AHAs Alpha Hydroxy Acids, also known as 'fruit acids' – including lactic, citric, malic, glycolic and tartaric acids – which brighten the complexion by loosening the bonds in the skin, helping to get rid of the flaky top layer and speeding up cell renewal.

Anaesthetic A drug – either applied to the skin in the form of a cream, or injected – which numbs the area to be treated.

Arnica A botanical remedy (from arnica montana, which grows at altitude), which is known for its anti-inflammatory properties. Can be applied as a cream or taken as a homoeopathic remedy.

Asymmetry A difference between two sides of the face – lopsidedness – or between individual elements like eyes, brows, ears. (Most people have naturally slightly asymmetric features, but in some individuals these are more pronounced.)

BOTOX® Short for Botulinum Toxin, which is administered by injection to smooth lines by temporarily paralysing the muscles that make specific expressions (like frowning). Can also be used as a treatment for sweating.

Bovine From cows. (As in: Collagen.)

BSE Bovine Spongiform Encephalopathy, or 'Mad Cow Disease'; fear of infection may be an anxiety for some patients undergoing collagen treatment.

Chemical peel The application of chemicals (usually acid) to peel away the upper layers of skin, revealing new, brighter layers underneath.

Contraindication Any illness, existing condition, allergy or disease that makes it risky to perform a procedure, take a particular drug or undergo a specific treatment. (NB It is extremely important to share a full medical history with the doctor/nurse/therapist who's carrying out any procedure, as even some natural, over-the-counter herbs – like St. John's Wort – may be 'contraindicated' for some treatments. The motto: better safe than sorry.)

Cadaver Dead person. (Some 'fillers' – such as Dermalogen, which is available in the US, among other places – use collagen derived from bodies, although some of this may come from procedures like breast reduction, after which women can opt to donate their tissue.)

Cannula/cannulae A thin, hollow tube which can be inserted under the skin and used to suck out fat under vacuum pressure (such as in liposuction, or the removal of fat for transplant elsewhere).

Collagen A natural element of human skin vital for tone, resilience and the 'bounce back' factor. (The collagen used in injections, however, is usually animal-derived – or donated by humans; see **Cadaver**.) NB Collagen also features as an ingredient in skin creams, but these cannot 'fill' the skin in the same way as an injection and it is generally used for its moisturising properties.

Collagen Instant Therapy The specific brand name of a particular type of cow-derived (bovine) collagen.

Cosmeto–dermatology The field of dermatology that relates to aesthetic procedures, rather than skin conditions like acne or rosacea.

Corrugator The muscle that causes the 'frown' lines between the brows.

Couperose Skin that flushes easily and is prone to broken veins – usually linked to sensitivity.

Crow's feet The wrinkles around the eyes, also known as 'laugh lines' (but not usually considered very funny!)

Dermabrasion Resurfacing of the skin using an abrasive substance or device to even out skin texture – almost like 'sanding' the skin so that the pits of acne scars, for instance, are less obvious. (NB See Microdermabrasion for the 'lunchtime' version of this.)

Dermis The layer of skin under the epidermis (see below) which functions as a supporting frame for the outer portion of the skin; it contains elastin, collagen, small blood vessels, nerve branches and lymphatics.

Elastin With collagen, elastin forms the connective tissue which supports the skin, giving it tone and plumpness.

Epidermis The top (outer) layer of skin, also known as the stratum corneum; this part of the skin is essentially dead by the time it reaches the surface.

Erythema Redness of the skin, the result of increased blood flow.

Excision Removal by cutting.

Exfoliant A substance (either chemical or grainy, in the form of salts/aluminium crystals etc), which sloughs off the top layer of skin.

Extrusion When an implant – for instance in the lips – starts to become visible or poke through the skin, either through movement of the implant or thinning of the skin.

Fibroblast A fibre-forming cell in the skin. (These get lazier as we get older.)

Free radicals 'Cellular terrorists' in the skin, these are highly unstable molecules created by our bodies when exposed to sunlight, pollution or when we're stressed, leading to cell breakdown – resulting in skin ageing and internal disease.

Horny layer The surface layer, where skin cells die off and are shed (aka stratum corneum).

Frontalis The forehead muscle that makes the brows move up and down, and contributes to the cross-ways wrinkles on the forehead.

Glabellar The area between the brows themselves. (Both these muscles are frequently targeted in BOTOX® injections.)

Glycolic acid An AHA 'fruit acid' used in facial peels, including superficial and very superficial peels.

Hyperpigmentation Darkening of the skin due to an excess of pigment (melanin), as in 'sun spots' (also known as age spots) and melasma, which is hormone-related and may be triggered by pregnancy or taking the Pill. Hyperpigmentation can also occur on darker (Asian and black) skins due to trauma – something as slight as picking a spot can leave a black mark.

Hypopigmentation When patches of the skin 'bleach out' because of a reduction of pigment (melanin) – a possible side effect of laser and light therapy.

Incision A surgical cut in the body.

Keloid An overgrowth of fibrous scar tissue that results in a raised scar rather than a depression, often found on darker skins.

Laser Short for Light Amplification by the Stimulated Emission of Radiation – a machine that gives off an intense beam of light, at a specific wavelength, which can be very precisely controlled and directed.

Lymphatic system The body's 'drainage network', whereby fluid is carried from the tissues into the bloodstream, to be flushed away.

Liposuction The removal of of fat from the body with a hollow instrument via a small incision, using suction power.

Marionette lines The vertical creases that run downwards from the sides of the mouth towards the jawline.

Microdermabrasion Gentle abrasion of the top layers of skin by blasting it with tiny particles to exfoliate dead cells, which are then vacuumed up.

Milia Raised white bumps on the skin – actually small cysts – which some women are vulnerable to, particularly under the eye and on the upper cheek area.

Nasal labial fold The crease that runs from the outer corners of the base of the nose to the corners of the upper lip.

Oedema Swelling, puffiness or fluid retention after treatment, surgery or inflammation.

Outpatient surgery Treatment in a clinic or surgery that does not require an overnight stay.

Phenol A highly concentrated peeling formulation used as part of a deep and invasive peel. (NB Definitely not a 'quick fix'.)

Photoageing Sun-related skin damage, resulting in wrinkles, fine lines, age spots etc.

Ptosis (say it 'toe-sis') – A term for drooping in eyelids (as well as other parts of the body), sometimes a side effect of BOTOX® treatment.

Rosacea A skin condition in which the face, nose, cheeks and forehead develop dilated (broken) blood vessels, redness, pimples and or occasional breakouts.

Salicylic acid A 'beta hydroxy acid' (BHA) found in some anti-ageing treatments.

Scar The legacy of skin damage – due to trauma (such as a cut, a graze or even squeezing a spot) – which leaves a pale and usually depressed mark. (See also Keloid.)

Silicone A highly controversial synthetic substance that is available in an injectable form to fill facial lines, among other uses.

Subcutaneous Under the skin.

SPF Short for Sun Protection Factor, and often followed with a number that acts as as a guide to the level of protection offered by the skin cream – an SPF15 would technically allow you to stay out in the sun fifteen times longer than it would usually take you to burn, before suffering the same damage. However, SPFs are tested in lab conditions that are far removed from the ways we use them in real life, and in actual use, deliver somewhere between one-half and one-third of the figure specified.

Sunblock A chemical and/or mineral-based cream designed to act as a barrier against the sun's rays. (See SPF.)

Telangiectasia Small thread veins, as found in the face.

Topical Applied to the skin (as in numbing creams, steroid creams etc).

Ultrasound The use of a particular frequency of soundwaves, creating an almost imperceptible vibration, which can be used in some anti-ageing techniques.

UVA The part of the spectrum of the sun's rays that causes long-term damage – think of 'UVAgeing'.

UVB The part of the spectrum of the sun's rays that causes shorter-term damage – i.e. burning and redness – think of 'UVBurning'.

Vermillion border The visible lip tissue, from the area where you'd put lipliner to the 'wet' bit just inside!

Resources

Medical resources

The British Association of Aesthetic Plastic
Surgeons
Royal College of Surgeons
35-43 Lincoln's Inn Fields
London WC2A 3PN
020 7831 5161
Website: www.baaps.org.uk

The British Association of Cosmetic Doctors
Dr Patrick Bowler
Court House Clinic
New Road
Brentwood
Essex CM14 4GD

The British Association of Plastic Surgeons
Royal College of Surgeons
35-43 Lincoln's Inn Fields
London WC2A 3PN
020 7831 5161
Website: www.baps.co.uk

The British Association of Dermatologists
19 Fitzroy Square
London W1T 6EH
020 7383 0266
Website: www.bad.org.uk

The British Medical Association
BMA House
Tavistock Square
London WC1H 9JP
020 7387 4499

Independent consultant

Wendy Lewis is one of the only independent
consultants who will refer you to the best
person for the treatments and cosmetic
surgery procedures you're interested in. She
divides her time between London and
Manhattan. For details of appointments, ring:

Wendy Lewis & Co.
15 Sloane Gardens
London SW1W 8EB
0870 7430 544
Website: www.wlbeauty.com
Email: wlbeauty@aol.com

The doctors

My thanks go to the following doctors. I
interviewed many other individuals and wish
I could list all of them, but space constraints
prevail.

Dr Tina Alster
2311 M Street NW
Suite 200
Washington DC 20037
USA
001 202 785 8855
Website: www.skinlaser.com
Email: talster@skinlaser.com

Dr Patrick Bowler
Court House Clinic
New Road
Brentwood
Essex
CM14 4GD
01277 203 000
Website: www.courthouseclinic.com

Dr Fredric Brandt
550 Biltmore Way
Coral Gables
FL 33134 USA
001 305 443 6606

Brian Coghlan FRCS
14 Devonshire Mews West
London W1G 6QE
020 7487 0480

Dr Alastair Carruthers
820-943 West Broadway
Vancouver
BC V5Z 4E1
Canada
001 604 714 0222

Dr Elisabeth Dancey
28 Winchester Street
London SW1V 4NE
020 7821 8257
Website: www.facemagic.co.uk
(Outline, Evolution, Face Magic)

Professor Nicholas J. Lowe
The Cranley Clinic
3 Harcourt House
19A Cavendish Square
London W1M 9AD
020 7499 3223

Dr Laurie J. Polis
Soho Integrative
62 Crosby Street
New York
NY 10012
001 212 431 1600

Mr Jan Stanek FRCS
101 Harley Street
London W1G 6AH
020 7487 4454

COLLAGEN
Inner Medical Ltd
Forest Court
Oaklands Park
Wokingham
Berkshire RG41 2QJ
0800 888000

NEW-FILL®
Medi-Phill
45 Phillimore Walk
London W8 7RZ
020 7937 2377
Website: www.phillimoreclub.com

BOTOX®, Neurobloc®, fillers and lips – the cheats

EVA FRASER
Videos, tapes and books available by mail
order from:
The Studio
St. Mary Abbots
Vicarage Gate
London W8 4HN
020 7937 6616

JOEY NEW YORK
Exclusive to House Of Fraser. Mail Order call
020 7963 2000

TRISH MCEVOY
Mail order: Harvey Nichols/020 7235 5000

VICTORIA VOGUE
Screenface 020 7221 8289
Website: www.screenface.com

The zappers

COOLTOUCH®
c/o Professor. Nicholas Lowe (See above)
Website: www.cooltouch.com
c/o Professor Nicholas Lowe (see above)

or:

COOLTOUCH®
90 85 Foothills Blvd
Roseville
CA95 747
USA 001 916 677 1975

NLITE™
London Day Surgery Centre
Gloucester House
Woodside Lane
London N12 8TP
020 8445 1199
Website: www.ldsc.co.uk

SOFTLIGHT™
45 Cheval Place
Knightsbridge
London SW7 1EW
020 7581 4499
Website: www.softlight.co.uk

The zappers – the cheats

ORIGINS
0800 731 4039

JOEY NEW YORK
(As above)

Vein hopes!

Professor Nicholas Lowe (see above)

Mr. John Scurr
Lister Hospital
Chelsea Bridge Road
London SW1 W8RH
020 7730 9563
Website: www.jscurr.com

DORNIER MEDILASE™
London Day Surgery Centre
Gloucester House
Woodside Lane
London N12 8TP
020 8445 1199
Website: www.ldsc.co.uk

Vein hopes! – the cheats

DERMABLEND
Mail order 02476 644 356
Enquiries 0800 085 6947

DERMAL K
Enquires: 020 8349 2000
Mail Order: 0845 673 2222
Website: www.dermalk.com

LAURA MERCIER
Harrods 020 7730 1234
Space NK 020 7727 8063
Mail order Space NK 0870 169 9999

JANE IREDALE
Mail order 0800 328 2467
Website: www.janeiredale.com

Smile, please...

Dr. Anthony Newbury
72 Harley Street
London W1G 7HG
020 7580 3168
Website: www.londonsmiles.com

Dr. Sunny Luthra
Capital Dental Care
298 Fulham Road
London W1G 7HG

General Dental Council
37 Wimpole Street
London W1G 8DQ
020 7887 3800

(They hold lists of specialists across the country)

Dentics
020 7937 9339

Smile, please... – the cheats

DENBLAN toothpaste:
Space NK 020 7727 8063
Space NK mail order 0870 169 9999

The peel thing

CRYSTAL CLEAR INTERNATIONAL
28 Rodney Street
Liverpool L12TQ
0870 593 4934
Website: www.crystalclear.co.uk

BIOSKIN-LAS
Biofarm Laser Skin Clinic
52 Lambs Conduit Street
London WC1 3LL
020 7242 5749

MD FORTE
Cosmeceuticals Ltd.
3 Swinborne Court
Basildon
Essex SS13 1QA
01268 724411

CELLABRASION™
Cosmeceuticals Ltd.
3 Swinborne Court
Basildon
Essex SS13 1QA
01268 724411

The peel thing – the cheats

CRYSTAL CLEAR®
(See above)

EVE LOM
Space NK 020 7727 8063
Space NK Mail Order 0870 169 9999

JOEY NEW YORK
(As before)

PHILO*SOPHIA
Space NK 020 7727 8063
Space NK mail order 0870 169 9999

Let there be light...

FOTOFACIAL™
The Advanced Harley Street Clinic
85 Main Road
Gidiea Park
Romford
Essex RM2 5EL
07000 560821
Website: www.epilight-int.com

PHOTOREJUVENATION
Merit House
The Hyde
Colindale
London NW9 5AB
020 8205 3481

PRO-FACIAL™
FocusLaser
The Clinic
118 Harley Street
London W1G 7JL
020 7486 7333
Website: www.focuslaser.co.uk

ENLIGHTEN
enlighten Information Office
Second Floor
Market Chambers
Cathedral Square
Peterborough PE1 1XW
0870 800 5063
Website: www.enlightenbeauty.co.uk

Let there be light... – the cheats
BENEFIT
09011 130 001
Website: www.benefitcosmetics.com

The beauty buzz
DIBITRON M TIME MACHINE
Dibi UK Limited
30 The Metro Centre
Britannia Way
Coronation Road
London NW10 7PA
020 8838 3858
E-mail: dibiuk@ukgateway.net
Website: www.dibicenter.it

CACI QUANTUM
C.A.C.I. International (for nearest salons)
11 Heath Street
Hampstead
London NW3 6TP
020 7431 1033
Website: www.caci-international.co.uk

ERP FACE MAGIC™
Dr. Elisabeth Dancey (As above)

FUTUR-TEC
CACI International
11 Heath Street
Hampstead
London NW3 6TP
020 7431 1033
Website: www.caci-international.co.uk

The beauty buzz – the cheats
MARK TRAYNOR LIFT
Screenface 020 7221 8289
Website: www.screenface.com

The überfacials
ACUPUNCTURE FACIAL
Yuki Umeguchi
Holmes Place Bodycare Clinic
188a Fulham Road
London SW10 9PN
020 7352 9169
Yuki Umeguchi direct: 020 8749 2781

ENDOLITE LIFT 6
Endolite UK Ltd.
5 Dee Road
Richmond
Surrey TW9 2JN
020 8332 0271

ENVIRON
UNIT 1
1000 North Circular Road
London NW2 7JP
020 8450 2020
Website: www.environ.co.za
Email: environuk@aol.com

HYDRADERMIE
Guinot
R Robson Ltd.
The Clock House
High Street
Ascot
Berkshire SL5 7HU
01344 873123
Website: www.rrobson.co.uk

REJUVANESSENCE™
Head Office
Belle Vue Lodge
91 Cheyne Walk
London SW10 0DQ
020 7352 8458

The überfacials – the cheats
LIZ EARLE
Liz Earle by Mail 01983 813 914

Index